MILADY'S

MILADY'S

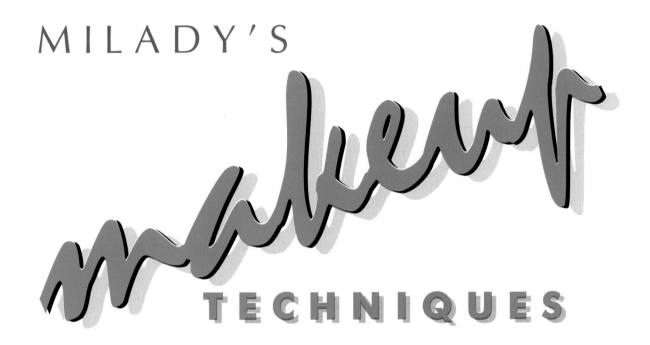

makeup

TECHNIQUES

00330112

PAMELA TAYLOR

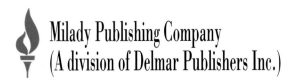

Milady Publishing Company
(A division of Delmar Publishers Inc.)

NOTICE TO THE READER

Publisher does not warrant or guarantee any of the products described herein or perform any independent analysis in connection with any of the product information contained herein. Publisher does not assume, and expressly disclaims, any obligation to obtain and include information other than that provided to it by the manufacturer.

The reader is expressly warned to consider and adopt all safety precautions that might be indicated by the activities herein and to avoid all potential hazards. By following the instructions contained herein, the reader willingly assumes all risks in connection with such instructions.

The Publisher makes no representation or warranties of any kind, including but not limited to, the warranties of fitness for particular purpose or merchantability, nor are any such representations implied with respect to the material set forth herein, and the publisher takes no responsibility with respect to such material. The publisher shall not be liable for any special, consequential, or exemplary damages resulting, in whole or part, from the readers' use of, or reliance upon, this material.

Milady Staff:
Publisher: Catherine Frangie
Developmental Editor: Joseph Miranda
Senior Project Editor: Laura Miller
Art & Production Manager: Susan Mathews
Freelance Project Editor: Pamela Fuller
Illustrator: Robert Richards
Cover Photographer: David Hamsley
Back Cover Photographer: Mychal Watts

Library of Congress Cataloging-in-Publication Data

Taylor, Pamela (Pamela Lynn), 1963-
    Makeup techniques / Pamela Taylor.
      p.   cm.
    ISBN 1-56253-142-5
    1. Cosmetics. 2. Beauty, Personal. I. Title.
RA778.T38   1993
646.7'2—dc20   93-25665
                                   CIP

DEDICATION

To my higher power and my wonderful mother and father —
thanks for giving me the gift of life.

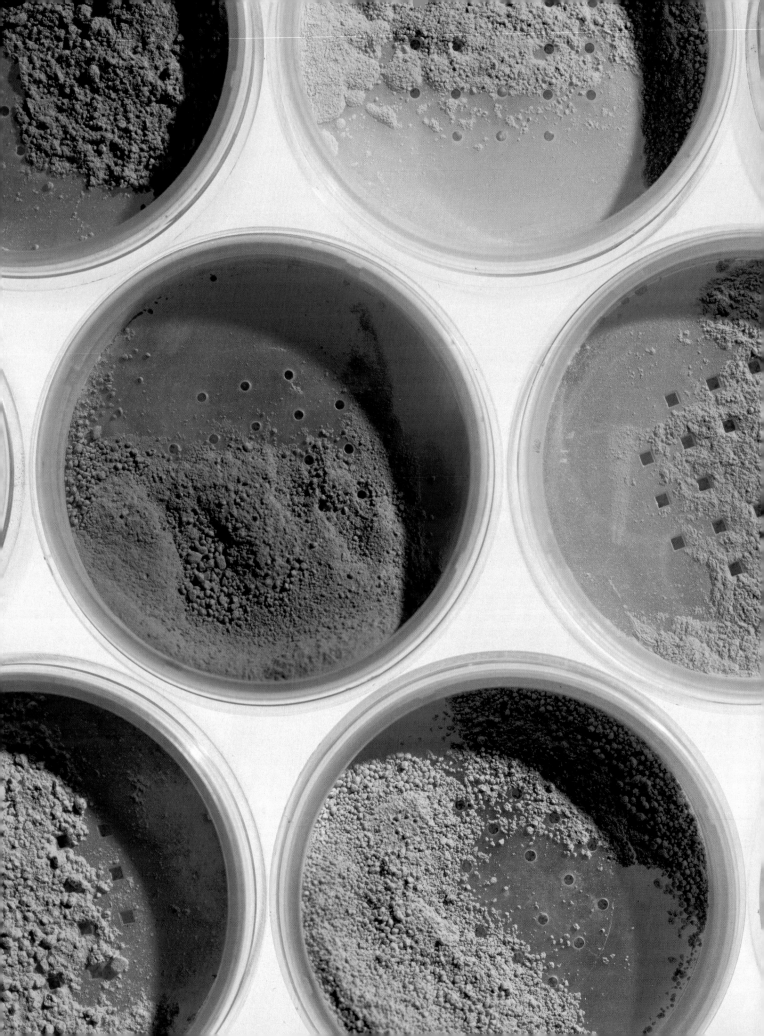

CONTENTS

PREFACE

Whether you are interested in the creative field of makeup artistry to improve your own appearance or as a career, I have written this book to share my professional knowledge with you. Through actual step-by-step photographs the world of professional makeup will be revealed in an easy-to-understand text, using behind-the-scenes techniques to create the remarkable look of models and celebrities in high-fashion magazines, in films, and on television. I hope my experiences will enable you to discover a most creative, exciting, and profitable career.

Reflecting on my childhood, I can clearly recall the interest I had in makeup since about the age of six. I remember shopping with my mom and how fascinating the colors, shapes, smells, and textures of makeup were. My favorite cartoon character was Penelope Pitstop, who had a pink convertible with an automatic lipstick dispenser built into the dashboard, and I loved Ginger on "Gilligan's Island," the movie star who was always creating changes with her makeup. As a child I never realized that a career in professional makeup was my destiny. As a young teenager, I recall feeling attracted to the beauty world, remembering magazine covers and scrutinizing every trace of color on the model, even noting who had done the makeup. I tried to imitate my favorite makeovers on my sisters and friends.

One day while in Manhattan, I passed by the Metropolitan Museum of Art. It was mesmerizing — a live model shoot with a photographer and a makeup artist! It was a vision of what I one day wanted to become. My high school guidance counselor also believed that a career in the beauty field would be my best choice. I attended cosmetology courses and graduated at the age of seventeen.

Afterwards I began my search and quest to learn professional makeup. There were only a few books available on the market, and not much information on this exciting and rewarding course of study. I then searched for a school and found only one available in the New York area. After completing the course I was convinced that the instructor should take a class herself. Determined to learn, I looked for a position in the field. After answering a help-wanted ad for a makeup artist consultant (will train) position, I was recruited to buy a makeup kit and attend a seminar with a man who probably has no idea of the impact he made on my life. I attended an eight-hour class with about seventy-five people and absorbed so much professional information it was like striking a gold mine. I received a certificate and after leaving that seminar came home with the tools and know-ledge to get me started.

Unfortunately the sales part of my training was not what I wanted. I was mainly interested in application, so I called a local modeling agency and began doing makeup for photo sessions. Through that position, I became an educator, teaching models to understand their facial structures, and by doing that I attained most of the technical knowledge that I will share in this book.

With the help of clients and students, I realized the need for educational material on makeup techniques. I was disappointed that I could not learn much more until I decided to call the top television studios in New York. I trained with Bob Kelly, who then offered a course in theatrical makeup. Bob was one of the most giving and sharing people in the industry; he encouraged me to go further in the field. Since then, my career has grown by leaps and bounds.

By the age of twenty-five I had traveled the United States as a platform educator and makeup artist for many beauty shows, had owned several makeup concessions, and had held the position of Director of Educational Marketing for several New York skin care and makeup companies. I currently work with many celebrities and models in the industry. I began writing when a beauty editor asked me to write an article on makeup. Little did I know that there was still such a void of technical information; one article led to more than thirty published articles within two years.

I currently own the Pamela Taylor Makeup Academy in New York City, where I teach the information I wish had been available to me when I got started. My hope is that if you have an interest in learning professional makeup, my book will teach you the tricks of the trade and the special ingredients necessary to become successful. Enjoy your learning experiences, you can never know too much! As you turn the pages of my book, may it turn the pages of your life.

Pamela Taylor
New York City

ACKNOWLEDGMENTS

- Jane Allen — Special thanks to my best friend, who through the years has encouraged me to go for my dreams. Your creative input and art direction helped to make the many hours of this project a pleasure.

- Kevin Mazur — To my favorite photographer and good friend. Although our busy schedules conflicted, and I unfortunately could not have your talent displayed in this book, your recommendations and input was greatly appreciated. P.S. Thanks for the ice cream!

- David Hamsley — seeing your work in *Glamour* magazine motivated me to find out who this great still life photographer was. A big thanks for all your precious time. P.S. I am glad we met, and yes you can make the squiggles.

- Thanks to all the bookers and models at the agencies in New York and Miami.

- Christian Pollard — to someone I really appreciate. Thank you for all the hours of casting, shooting, and computer lessons; your effort and talent was immeasurable.

- Barbara Jewett — Thank you for recommending me to write this book. You are an incredible editor and a lovely person — many sincere thanks.

- Greg Lewis — thanks for your encouragement.

- N.G., M.S., J.M., L.V., C.C., and all the cosmetology teachers who have always encouraged me to excel, may your positive influence and teaching skills inspire many others to succeed.

- To my "always on the go" editor Catherine Frangie, thank you for your patience and understanding. P.S. Cathy, I think we need a cruise!

- To the man who always has a smile — Joe Miranda, my project coordinator and editor, thanks for your input.

- Terry Beuchamp — thanks for helping with the book; you will never be forgotten!

- To all my family, friends, colleagues, professors, and former students, who through years of experiencing life made it possible for me to gain the knowledge to write a book, thank you for your support.

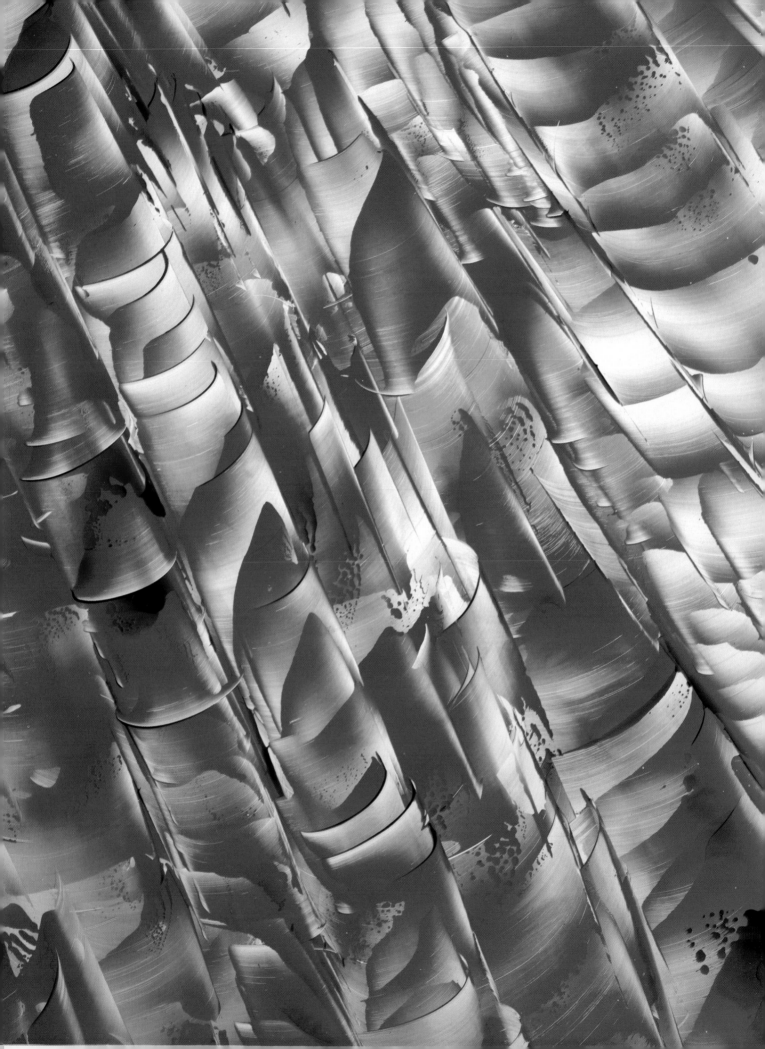

INTRODUCTION TO MAKEUP ARTISTRY

Welcome to the exciting and profitable world of professional makeup. Although there are several beautiful makeup books on the market, they didn't include professional makeup techniques in photographic detail with a variety of live models of different ethnic types.

This book is packed with the techniques and information you will need to achieve the confidence in order to apply makeup like a professional. The detailed photography, beautiful illustrations, and easy-to-comprehend subject matter make this book an essential addition to your makeup library. This book is designed as an educational tool, and it provides such detail that anyone wanting to learn makeup application can comprehend and apply the technical information provided to achieve flawless makeup applications for professional or personal use.

As you turn the pages, you will view the secrets that have made my makeup techniques so successful. You will notice that we went to the fullest extent to demonstrate hand dexterity, and each tool is captured in step-by-step photographs, demonstrating the proper application techniques that are essentials for makeup applications.

The actual samplings of each color palette have been photographed — in lifelike detail.

Although the trends in fashion are constantly changing, this book will provide you with the most important application techniques, which will never change. I encourage anyone who is craving knowledge in makeup application to read and comprehend this easy-to-follow book of makeup techniques.

prior to...

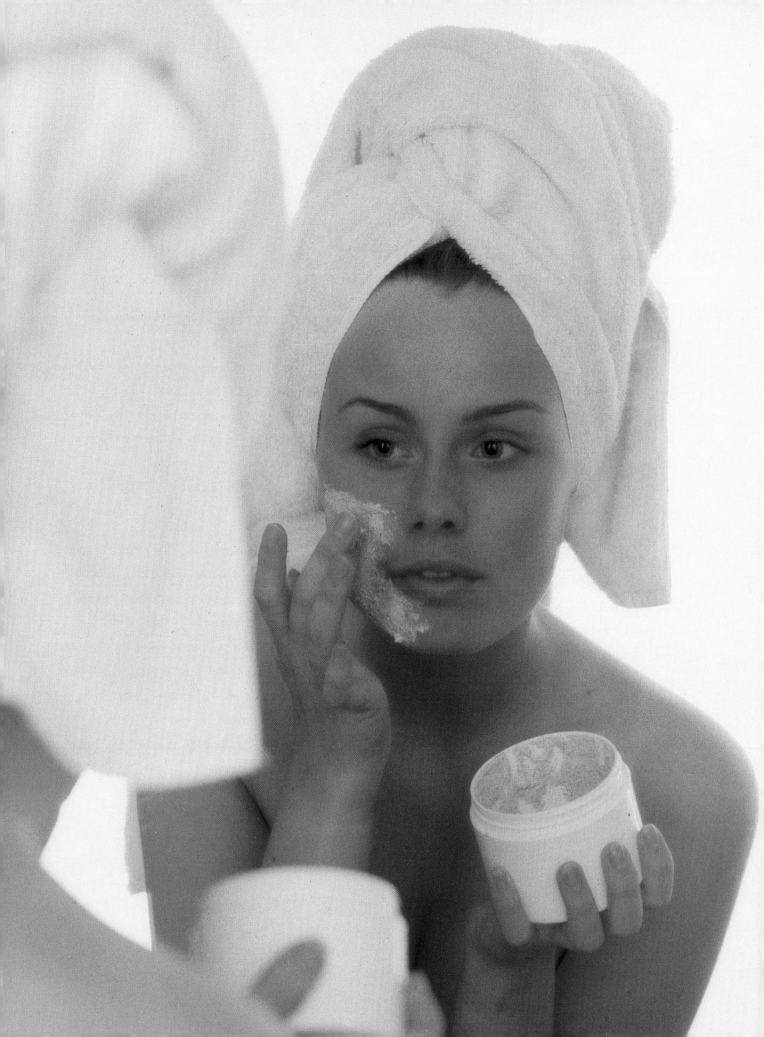

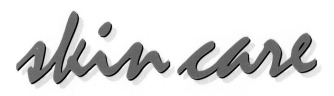

skin care

BEFORE APPLYING MAKEUP...

Although you are not giving a facial, it is important to take a few moments to properly care for the skin. In my kit I carry a cleanser, toner, and protective moisturizer for all skin types, including normal, dry, and oily skin.

As a professional makeup artist, I have learned through hands-on experience how important it is to care for the delicate and precious skin on the face. Although we cannot stop the aging process, caring for the skin (meaning eating a nutritious diet, regular exercise, minimal stress, avoiding weather extremes, and protecting the skin from excessive sun exposure) will help keep your face in its best possible condition. It is important to note that for severe conditions of dryness, acne, or unusual looking skin lesions, it is best to recommend the treatment of a dermatologist prior to concealing the problem with makeup products.

The following are three steps for skin preparation on all skin types. Select a product line for your skin type; then apply the three steps. Keep in mind that you are not conducting an entire facial, and the time spent on basic skin care should be minimal.

I enjoy using a natural product line on myself and my clients. Several excellent skin-care lines are available on the market. I recommend consulting a professional esthetician or makeup artist who is knowledgeable about the most effective products available.

Step 1

Cleanse the face using a cream cleanser on a moistened cotton pad. Always apply cleanser in an upward motion, repeating the procedure until all signs of residue are gone. Do not forget the neck and ear areas. In addition, when working around the mouth, make sure to remove lipstick inward toward the center of the mouth to avoid staining the surrounding facial skin.

When cleansing around the eyes, remove mascara by closing the eye and using a cotton pad moistened with eye makeup remover. Sweep the pad downward over the lashes, then inward toward the inner corners of the eye. It is important never to pull or stretch the delicate skin in this area. Always check to see if your client is a contact lens wearer, and if the client is sensitive to the product you are using.

Step 2

You may rinse the face with room temperature water. Then apply a toner to a cotton pad, gently working upward toward the forehead to balance, freshen, and remove excess residue on the skin.

Step 3

Protect the skin using a moisturizer that will help to create a barrier between the makeup and the skin. No matter what the skin type, a protective moisturizer is a necessity prior to makeup application because of its ability to help any liquid or cream based products blend more effectively.

PROFESSIONAL TIPS

Drink six to eight glasses of water daily. Water helps to hydrate the skin as well as flush out many toxins. Avoid a high salt or alcohol intake; this will dehydrate the skin and cause it to look unhealthy.

Avoid using soap, unless you can find a soap that is not harsh on the skin. Soap has the ability to strip the skin of its natural oils and leaves the skin feeling tight with residue or film. Even on oily skin, soap is not recommended unless it is pH balanced.

Deep clean the skin at least once a month. Treat yourself to a professional facial or a facial at home. I believe in holistically based skin-care and facial treatments; facials help to stimulate the skin and clean the pores of excess residue from environmental pollutants.

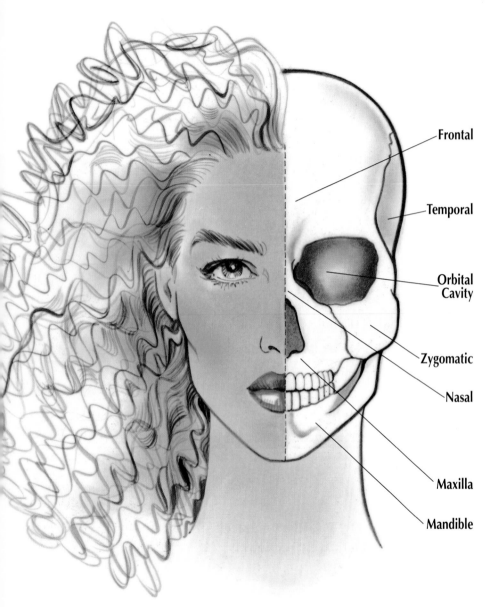

Frontal

Temporal

Orbital
Cavity

Zygomatic

Nasal

Maxilla

Mandible

Analyzing the bone structure will help you determine what areas should be emphasized or de-emphasized prior to applying makeup to the face. By using the skillful application of contours (darker shades) and highlights (paler shades), facial features can appear altered or enhanced. To determine the facial shape of a client, it is important to become familiar with the following bones of the head and face.

❏ Frontal bone — forms the forehead.

❏ Temporal bones — form the sides of the head in the ear region.

❏ Zygomatic or molar bones — form the prominence of the cheeks.

❏ Nasal bones — form the bridge of the nose.

❏ Lacrimal bones — small fragile bones located at the front part of the inner wall of the eye sockets.

❏ Maxillae bones — upper jawbones which join to form the whole upper jaw.

❏ Mandible — lower jawbone. It is the largest and strongest bone of the face and forms the lower jaw.

highlights

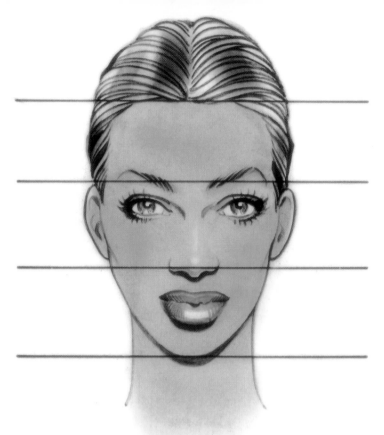

Although there are several other bones that form the anatomy of the head and face, it is the above named bones that are important to know when studying a client's facial shape and deciding what parts to highlight or de-emphasize with makeup.

For many years, the rule has been that the so-called "ideal face" shape is the oval face. Using the oval as a guideline, you can determine a person's face shape by referring to any areas that fall inside or outside the guide. This is an easy way to learn face shapes and is not intended to teach you that every face should be oval shaped.

To me what makes a face unique is the bone structure. The only time I suggest altering the appearance of the face is when an area or feature is distracting. Looking at the profile of the face, the forehead and chin should be vertically balanced, and from a straight-on view, the start of the hairline to the inner brow, the brow to the base of the nose, and the base of the nose to the chin should be in proportion. Knowing the shape and size of the area you are working on will help you determine whether you will contour or highlight the feature.

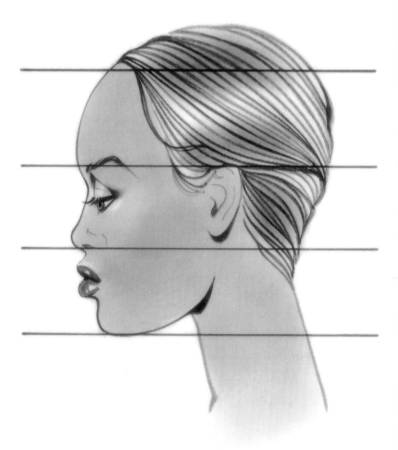

Contouring products are available in liquid (a deeper shade of foundation), powder, and cream formulas. Contouring products are used to recede areas of the face and should be deeper, matte shades ranging from soft taupe to deep ash brown.

Highlighting products are light reflective and can range from bright pearly whites to matte beige shades. The main purpose of using highlights is to bring facial features forward so they appear larger or fuller. Highlights are available in cream, powder, and liquid formulations.

Contouring and highlighting products should be applied following the foundation or when priming the canvas of the face prior to color.

When applying contouring and highlighting products, avoid harsh lines of demarcation and keep placement of products detailed and concentrated to the area where the change is desired.

Knowing the bone structure can help determine if an area is "out of proportion" to the facial structure, and working with the natural architecture of the face, the makeup artist can alter the appearance by using the corrective procedures described below.

FOREHEAD

Wide — apply a shading product to the outer corners and blend toward the hairline.

Small or short — highlight the center of the forehead to open the area.

Protruding — apply shading over the area to make the forehead appear to recede.

High — apply shading around the edge of the forehead and blend back toward the hairline.

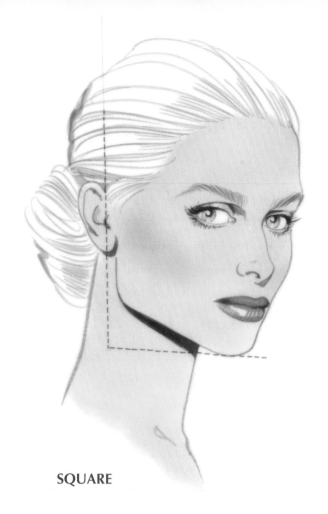

SQUARE

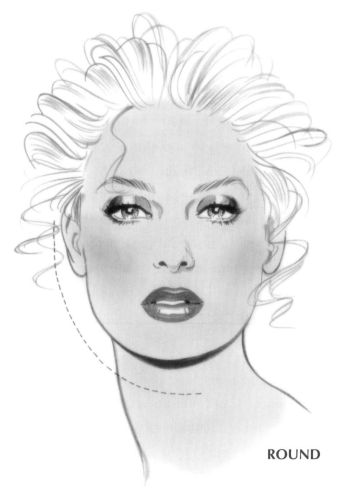

ROUND

CHEEKBONES

Long or flat — to create the illusion of width, apply highlighting to both sides of the face horizontally above the natural bone. Apply blush using the guideline created on the cheek area below.

Too full and round — apply contouring beneath the natural cheekbone hollow to create a thinner appearance. Highlight near the temple and upper part of the cheekbone to achieve an angular appearance.

Low — apply highlighter to the upper, outer part of the cheekbone in an angular line to lift the area. Choose a lighter cheek color beneath the highlighter.

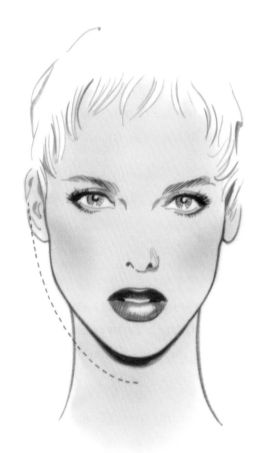

OVAL

JAW

Square — for a very broad jaw, apply contouring or a deeper shade of foundation at the squared corners to soften the line; blend well and make sure not to create a line of demarcation.

Narrow — to create a fuller appearance in the outer area of the jaw, apply highlighting at both sides of the jaw and blend.

Uneven — You can either contour or highlight the side of the face that is out of proportion. If one side of the jaw is more prominent, simply apply shading to the area that protrudes and blend to soften. You can then highlight the opposite side to create balance.

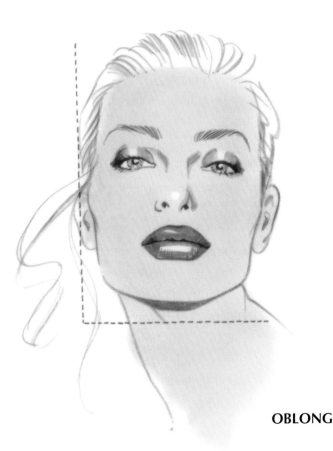

OBLONG

CHIN

Pointed — shade the tip of the chin; then highlight the outer corners of the jaw to create the illusion of balance. Blend well.

Receding — simply apply highlighting to the tip of the recessed area and blend well.

Large, squared tip — soften the edges of the chin at the outer corners; then blend.

Double chin — apply shading to the recession of the jawbone; then shade over the heaviest area to lift the chin. (This is detailed and should be carefully applied.)

Long — apply shading over the most prominent area; then blend.

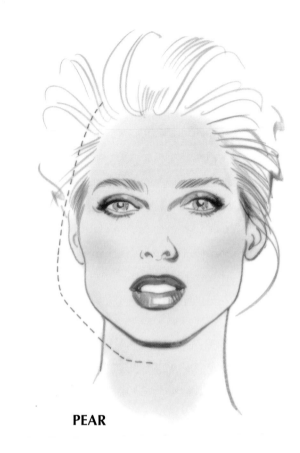

PEAR

NOSE

Wide — shade the sides and blend back toward the face, then lighten the center of the bridge of the nose.

Rounded tip — shade the edges of the round tip to create a softer appearance.

Long — shade the tip of the nose to give a shorter appearance.

Uneven nostrils at the base of the nose — lighten the higher part of the nostril or darken the lower area to create balance.

Bump — darken the most prominent part of the bump and blend to recede the area.

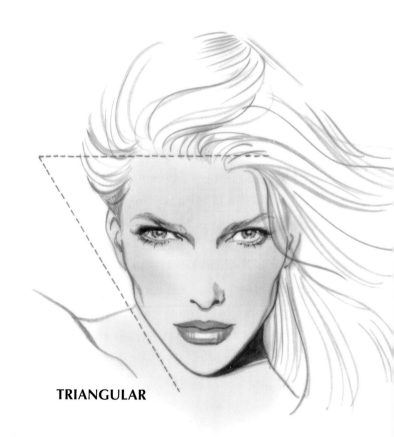

TRIANGULAR

Uneven nose — apply two straight lines of contour directly.

Turned-up or pug-style nose — darken the upper tip of the area.

The corrective procedures described above can be used to correct most facial shapes. The most common shapes are illustrated on pages 20 - 23, and shading has been applied to illustrate the area where the change is needed. To contour and highlight the lips or eyes, refer to their sections indicated in the book.

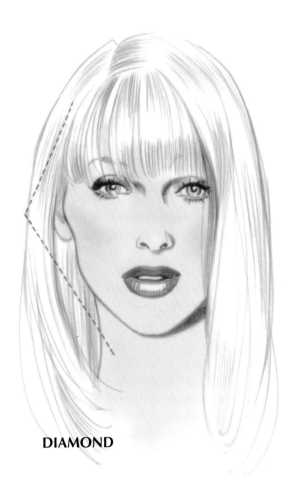

DIAMOND

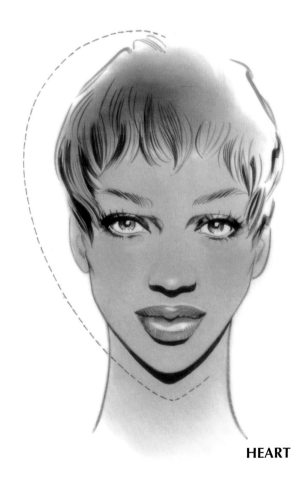

HEART

hand dexterity

Proper hand dexterity is one of the most important yet overlooked aspects of makeup application. To the best of my knowledge, the subject of hand dexterity has never been explained in any depth. Nevertheless, its importance cannot be overestimated. Just as an artist uses a strong or subtle touch of the hand or stroke of the brush to create a soft or dramatic image, so a makeup artist uses the hand and brush on the canvas of the face to create a desired effect.

Before beginning the makeup application, make sure the client is sitting with the head more or less at your eye level. I recommend a director's chair or a hydraulic chair with a comfortable back. Not only does this avoid back strain, enabling you to work more comfortably, but you can view the face at eye level. Looking down on a face creates shadows. Second, position yourself as close as comfortable to the subject's body so you can see exactly what you are doing and so you can gain more control. Do not apply makeup from a distance further than the distance between your elbow and your client's shoulder.

One of the most important reasons for good hand dexterity is that it conveys a sense of security to the client, who can feel the makeup artist's confident touch.

The physiology of hand dexterity begins with an understanding of how the movements of the shoulder, arm, elbow, hand, and fingers coordinate to apply proper pressure and direction to your makeup tools. Think of your tools as extensions of your body. Just as a finely tuned athlete knows how to use the body to achieve a desired result — whether swinging a bat or handling a ball — so too will your understanding of how the body works together and how it will affect your final results help you use your body effectively.

TECHNIQUES

Relax. Relax. Relax.

The Shoulder

Think of your shoulder as a pivot. The shoulder controls the amount of pressure on your tools. It is extremely important not to put your entire body weight behind your movements when applying makeup, but to isolate these movements from the shoulder. Remember not to lean into your client, since this can cause discomfort. Maintain a balanced posture, and you will maintain better control.

The Elbow

Think of your elbow as a guide. All motion in the forearm is controlled by the elbow. When applying makeup, the elbow is positioned slightly below the shoulder.

Application

When touching the face, always be prepared to pull away. Apply light, featherlike touches to the delicate facial skin. Never apply excess pressure to the face. It causes discomfort and overapplication of product to the face. Never use full force from your arm; practice gently touching the face and becoming aware of the weight you apply to the face.

EXERCISES

To help control your movements, practice the following exercises. Hold the hand in a straight line from the elbow to the wrist; then practice moving the forearm back and forth or up and down on the face, applying gentle pressure to the face. This is one method of blending when holding a wedge or powder puff.

Or use a rolling, side-to-side or back-and-forth motion for blending shadows. When holding an eyeshadow brush or applicator, I recommend holding the brush the same way you would hold a pencil; this will allow you to control the application in a small, detailed area.

When you apply foundation using a wedge or a sponge, use feather-light hand motions. Come from the shoulder, keep a fluid motion, and relax your wrist. Use long, downward strokes. Start at the forehead; use long strokes, taking care not to apply too much pressure. Think of frosting a chocolate cake with vanilla frosting.

Blush and loose powder application requires similar wrist movements as used in applying shadow. For blush application, following the line of the natural cheekbone, start at the outer part of the face and, keeping the elbow stationary, blend forward by turning the wrist smoothly in a clockwise direction. Hold the powder brush and blend over the entire face using a gentle touch.

For the lips, work against the muscle by applying the lip pencil or lip brush starting at the outer corner of the mouth and moving up toward the center. The tautness will aid in an easier, more even application procedure. You can rest the pinky finger on the chin for balance while holding the brush or pencil as you would hold a writing pencil.

When applying makeup, observe the hand motions you are using to apply the makeup. Keep consistent in your work, and remember that a professional makeup application should be a relaxing experience for the client. After practicing and mastering hand dexterity, you will more than likely be complimented on your confident and relaxing touch.

A well-stocked, professional looking makeup kit is an essential for the makeup artist. A professional makeup kit should stock a range of colors and a variety of products to handle all skin types and tones. In my kit, I carry a variety of makeup products and tools to handle virtually any job. Keeping your kit well organized and clean is also very important. I have seen many makeup artists ruin their

images by arriving at a job with a shopping bag full of makeup that is dirty and unorganized. This reflects the way they usually will work, in a disorganized and unsanitary manner. Pictured is my professional kit, which I use for most of the beauty photo shoots and

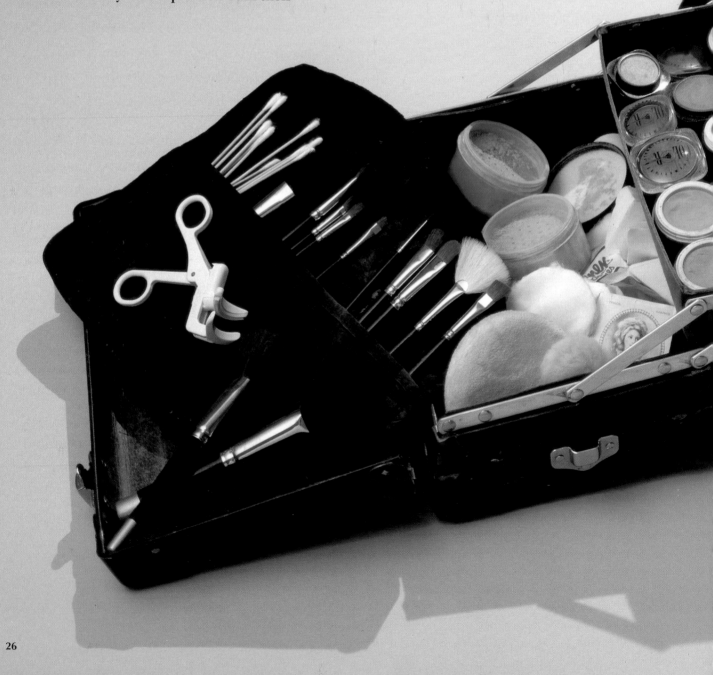

makeup kit

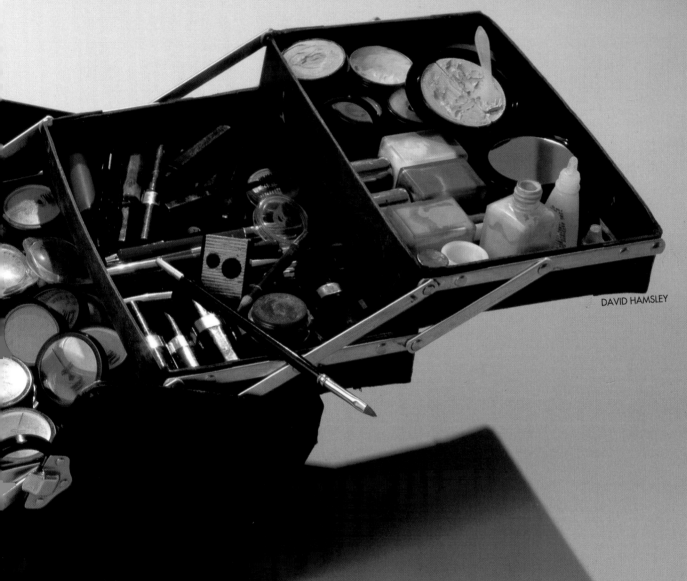

DAVID HAMSLEY

many makeup artists in the industry, and it is convenient for the artist on the go. I travel extensively with my kit, and it is made to withstand much use. If you are arranging a kit for personal use, many similar cases are available that are constructed from molded plastics. Whether you are arranging a personal makeup collection for at home, or preparing a kit for professional use, most of the items suggested on the following pages should be included.

makeovers I do. In addition, I have a theatrical kit, which contains a range of special effect makeup products. It is evident that although my kit is well used, I keep it neat and organized. The kit pictured is a three-tiered, custom-made case. This type of case is used by

SUPPLIES

Tissues

Tissues are convenient to use as a blotting tool for removal of excess moisturizer or for sifting powder through onto the lipstick (see lip application techniques). They can also be used beneath the eye as a powder guard, folded to keep shadows from falling onto the face. I do not recommend using tissues to clean the face; they tend to be too abrasive for the delicate facial skin.

Cotton

Cotton is available in rolls or squares. Pure, natural, 100 percent cotton has several uses and is recommended for use prior to and during the application process. Loose rolled cotton must be pulled from the roll and folded at the corners, then moistened in water and pressed to remove excess water. This technique is used by many skin-care experts and is most economical. The corners must be rolled to eliminate loose pieces of stray cotton on the face; according to the desired size you can alter the rolled cotton to your liking.

Cotton squares or rounds are pre-formed, pressed cotton applicators, usually sold in a dispensable bag, and are excellent for blotting excess makeup and pressing makeup onto the face. Cotton is the recommended fiber to use for all cleansing and hydrating procedures.

Cotton swabs are excellent disposable tools for erasing mistakes and cleaning hard-to-reach areas of the face. To quickly remove unwanted makeup such as mascara or uneven lipliner, dip a tightly wound cotton swab into a small amount of cream, then twirl onto the area that needs to be "lifted" and watch how the swab removes the product. You can clean hard-to-reach eye corners and lip corners; swabs may also be used to apply powder to the ears to reduce shine in photographic makeup. I recommend using surgical cotton swabs; they are rolled tightly onto a long wooden applicator, are flexible and easy to work with, and are available at most pharmacies. In the event that you can not locate them, you can make your own by wrapping rolled cotton around an orangewood stick.

Brushes

In order to achieve the best possible blending and application results, quality brushes must be used. (see the Tools of the Trade section)

Skin-care Products

Carry a selection of cleansers, toners, and protective face lotions for all skin types. I recommend storing skin-care products in portable size containers for on the go use.

Headband

Disposable cotton fiber bands are available in roll form. This type of band is gentle on the hair and will fit any head size. Miss Webril brand hair wraps are available at most beauty suppliers and are an excellent choice.

Hand Sanitizer

A hand sanitizer, available in pump form, quickly cleans and sanitizes the hands and comes in scented formulas to remove any offensive odors.

Liquid Brush Cleaner

Quickly removes color from the brush and dries within a minute or two. Brushes should be cleaned and sanitized between each client.

An ultraviolet ray sanitizer is recommended for a busy location (a salon or a store) to keep implements and tools sterilized and free of germs and bacteria.

Makeup Collection

❏ Concealers

❏ Foundation (all types)

❏ Contouring/shading products

❏ Highlighting products

❏ Face powders — loose/pressed

❏ Blushers — a variety of shades and formulas

❏ Eyeshadows — a variety of warm, cool, matte, and pearl colors

❏ Eye contouring pencils and brow pencils

❏ Lipsticks and glosses — a variety of colors in tube, pot, and wand formulas

❏ Liplining pencils

❏ Assorted artificial lashes, strip and individual

❏ Eyelash glue — clear

❏ Mascara — assorted formulas and colors

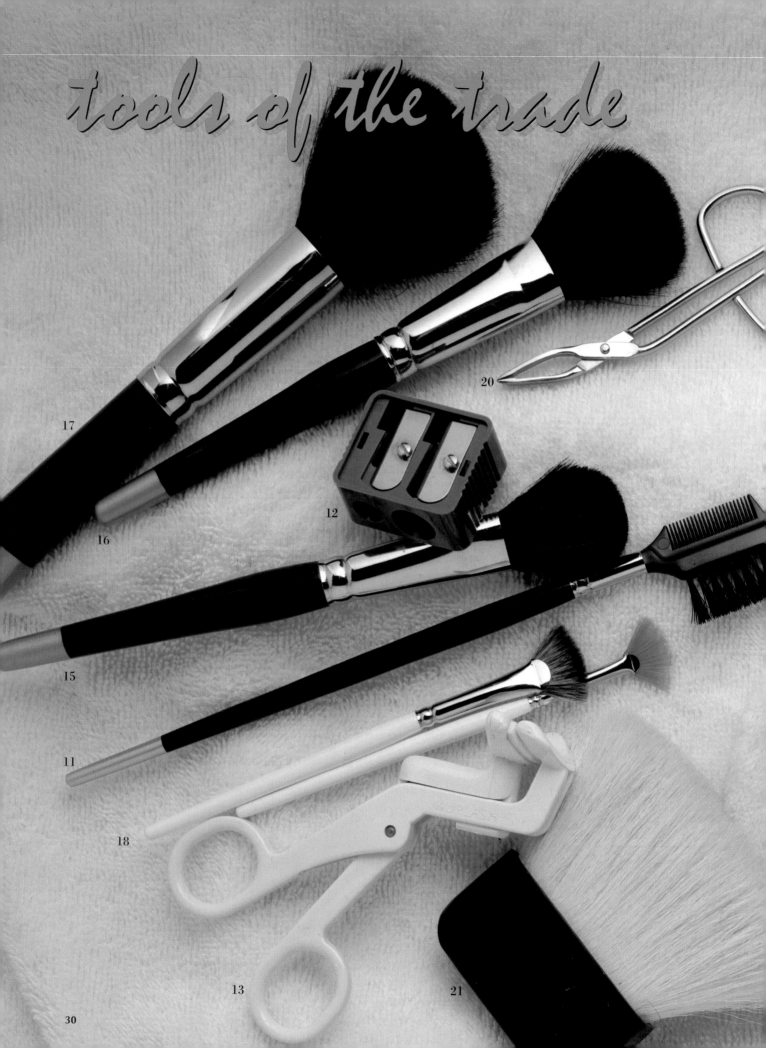

tools of the trade

20

17

16

12

15

11

18

13

21

30

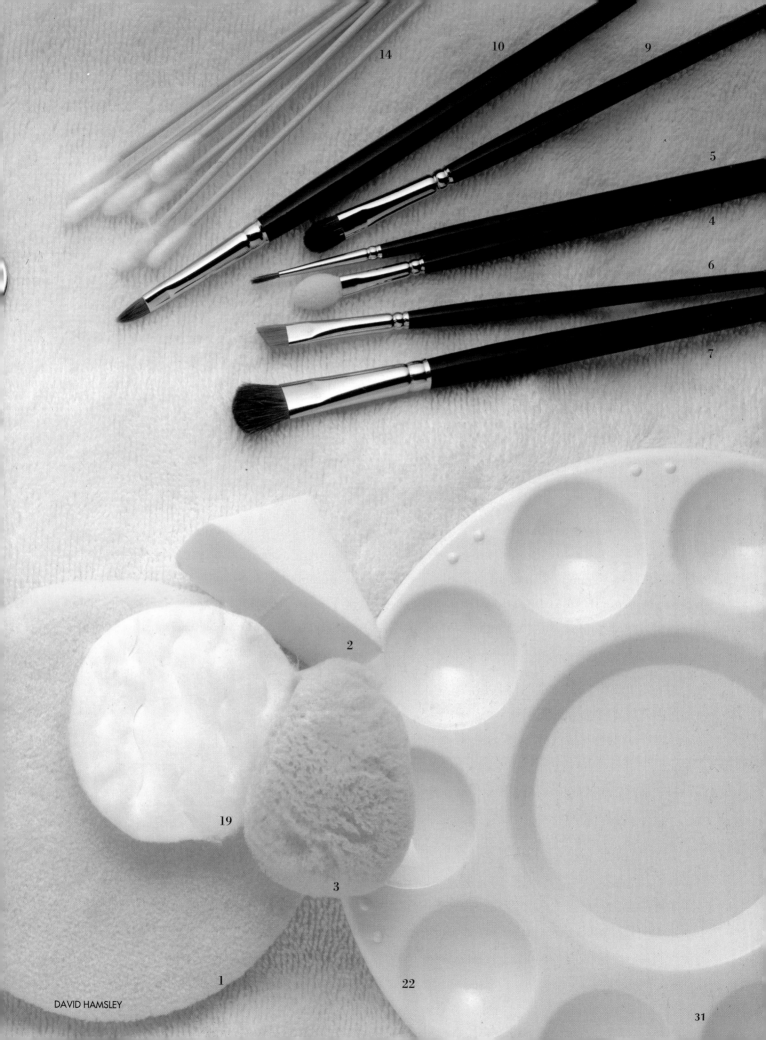

14
10
9
5
4
6
7
2
19
3
1
22

DAVID HAMSLEY

31

Professional tools are an important addition to the makeup artist's kit. Working with the best quality tools will assure you optimal results. Many tools are available on the retail market, and it can sometimes become confusing deciding what to look for when selecting the proper tools for your makeup kit. Although brushes are manufactured with both synthetic and natural hair, I recommend a selection of natural bristle brushes for use in your kit.

Powder, blush, lip, and shadow brushes should be constructed with a strong metal furrow (the metal attachment that secures the brush hairs). The furrow is crimped according to the shape of the brush. For example, when a narrow, tapered, angular, shadow brush is constructed, the metal is crimped very tightly to create a flat base for the hair. Some brushes on the market are constructed using aluminum for the furrow. I do not recommend purchasing this type of brush — the metal usually bends, resulting in an awkward brush shape. The best metal to look for is chrome-plated brass, which is both durable and attractive.

Brush handles are another important consideration when choosing a brush — they are available in plastic, metal, or wood. The handle helps achieve balance when applying makeup; therefore the length and shape of the handle are important considerations. Unlike plastic or metal brush handles, which are usually constructed in awkward shapes and sizes, opt for a wooden handle that is rounded and tapered at both ends. Usually this type of brush can be found through an artist's supply store or a professional beauty source. Handle lengths range from 3 to 6 inches; I personally prefer using a 6-inch handle, which is the choice of most professional makeup artists. The longer handle allows lighter hand dexterity and better balance during makeup application.

Proper maintenance of makeup brushes is the best way to ensure longer lasting tools and sanitary makeup application. Often I apply makeup to a large group of models in a short time period, and to use a new set of brushes for each model would be virtually impossible. Not only would this take up too much room in my kit, it would become very costly. Fortunately there is an alternative to the soap and water method of cleaning brushes. There is a professional brush cleaner, available where many professional beauty supplies are sold, that dries in about one minute and sterilizes the brushes between each use. However, I recommend cleaning the natural bristle brushes regularly by immersing them in warm sudsy water, using a mild detergent and then rinsing until clean. Dry the brushes end up in a jar and reshape when they are completely dry. Never blow dry brushes; the hair will frizz and break, and the heat will contract the wooden handle.

SELECTION OF TOOLS

The following tools are shown, with the corresponding numbers, on pages 30 and 31. (Brushes courtesy of Silver Tip, New York City)

1. Velour Powder Puff — These are available in a variety of sizes. They are used to press powder onto the face and offer a

concentrated amount of product; they are best used with loose face powder. (Never pull across the skin; gently press over the makeup to set and to remove excess shine.)

2. Sponge Wedge — A pie-shaped sponge usually constructed of latex, that is used to apply and blend makeup. Use the flat sides to apply foundation and the corners to get into hard-to-reach areas. Can be used dry or moistened. A good quality wedge simulates the pores of natural skin and will expand when wet.

3. Natural Sea Sponge — This sponge can be used to apply foundation, has a soft, silky texture, and is ideal for body makeup. Using it can sometimes result in a streaky appearance if it is not used properly.

4. Chamois Applicator — This applicator is constructed of sheepskin; it is long lasting, soft, and ideal for applying concealer to the undereye area. It is not recommended for eyeshadows, because the cloth will hold the color.

5. Fine Eyeliner Brush — A gradually tapered pointed brush for use in applying cake or liquid eyeliners; it is ideal for fine, detailed eyeliner.

6. Angular Shadow Brush — A tightly crimped angled brush that is used to apply eyeshadow at the base of the eyelids; it is also ideal for shaping and coloring the brows.

7. Small Fluff Brush — This is used to apply eyeshadow to the lids; it is very good for detailed application.

8. Large, Chiseled Fluff Brush — This brush is used to apply color to the contours of the eyes and also for blending shadows. (not pictured)

9. Small Blender Brush — This brush is ideal for applying highlighter to small

areas and also for buffing powder in hard-to-reach areas.

10. Chiseled Lip and Concealer Brush — This brush allows application of cream makeup and lip colors in small, detailed areas.

11. Brow Brush/Comb — This brush is used to brush the eyebrow hair and to separate lash hairs.

12. Duo Pencil Sharpener — A double sided sharpener is used for both thick and thin lip and eye pencils.

13. Eyelash Curler — This is used to curl the upper lashes prior to mascara application.

14. Surgical Cotton Swab — A swab is used to clean up mistakes and to remove excretions from the corners of the eyes and lips.

15. Chiseled Blush Brush — This brush is used for applying powdered cheek color.

16. Powder Brush — This brush is used for applying pressed or loose powder, to set makeup, or to remove excess shine from the face.

17. Large Powder Brush — A large brush is used for applying powder to large areas, the chest and shoulders.

18. Goat Fan Brush — A brush that is ideal for holding under the eyes while applying shadows; it catches excess color.

19. Cotton Pledget — This is used to remove makeup.

20. Tweezers — Use a fine quality, slanted, type to remove unwanted hair.

21. Body Blender — Use for blending body makeup.

22. Artist's Mixing Palette — A palette is used to mix color and store creams and water while working.

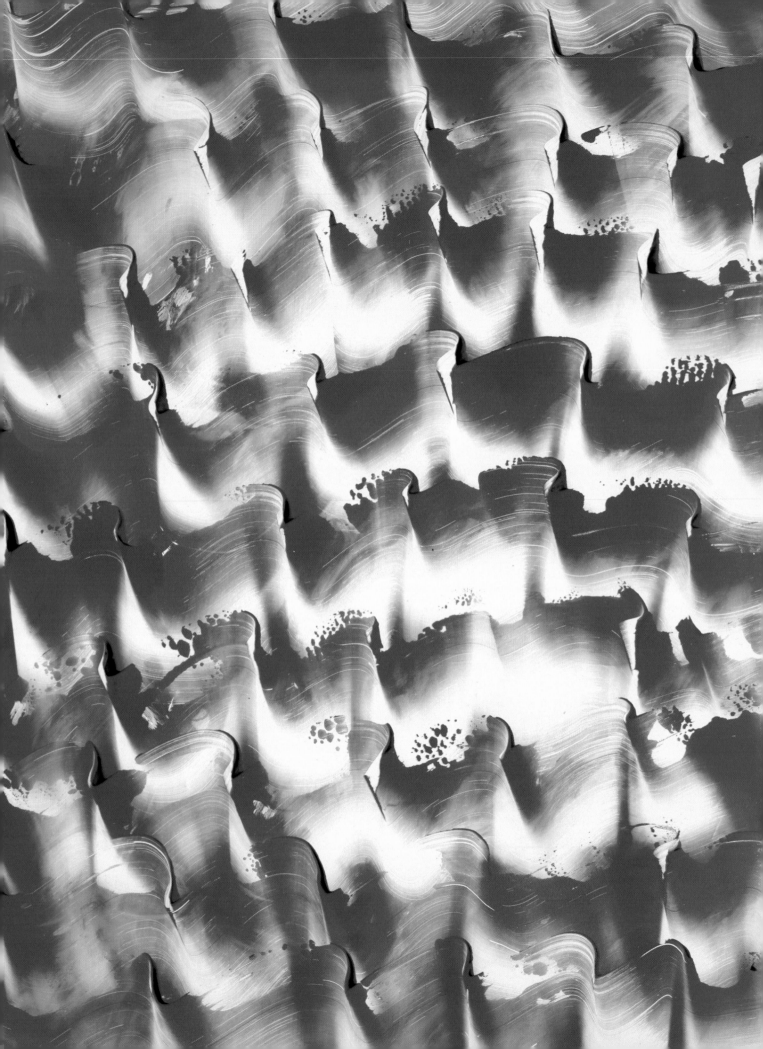

color

The most rewarding part of experimenting with make-up is the variety of color choices that you can work with. The look you create depends entirely on the palette you choose for the makeup application. No choice of color is "cut in stone" for any skintone or eye color, and the artistic and creative aspect of being a makeup artist allows you the freedom to choose and combine colors that best enhance a client's natural coloring.

I suggest studying the color wheel to gain an understanding of how color works, then, using skillful application techniques, begin to experiment with color to create a variety of looks with makeup. To create softer looks, choose softer, diffused shades of color in the warm or cool color spectrum.

For bolder, cleaner looks, you can choose brighter, clearer, or bolder colors. Colors can be placed beside each other to enhance or brighten or can be applied in softer hues to result in a monochromatic look. A variety of colors will help features such as the eyes "come alive" or can distract from or soften areas. As with any form of art, your personal style and choice of color will help to develop a style in your work. Remember to blend well and refer to the guidelines in the previous chapters on selecting foundation color. As far as color is concerned, the selection depends entirely on the effect you wish to portray.

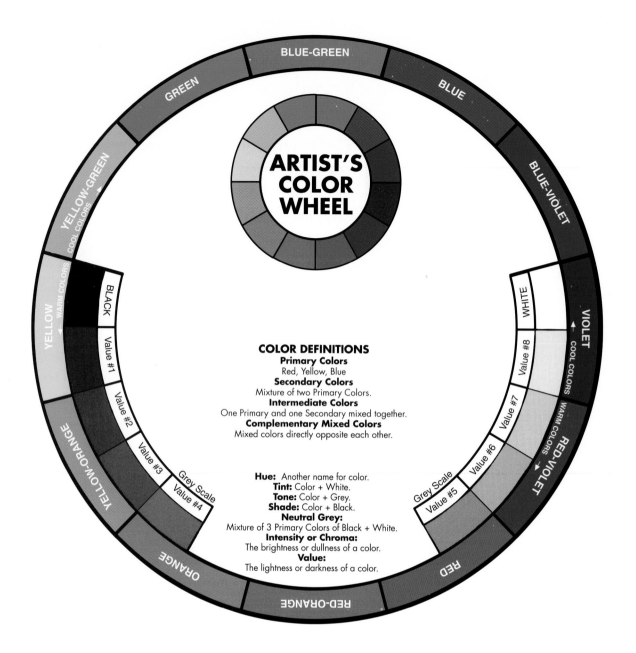

ARTIST'S COLOR WHEEL

BLUE-GREEN
GREEN
BLUE
YELLOW-GREEN
BLUE-VIOLET
COOL COLORS
VIOLET
YELLOW
WARM COLORS
COOL COLORS
WARM COLORS
RED-VIOLET
BLACK
WHITE
Value #1
Value #8
Value #2
Value #7
YELLOW-ORANGE
Value #3
Value #6
RED-VIOLET
Grey Scale
Value #4
Grey Scale
Value #5
ORANGE
RED
RED-ORANGE

COLOR DEFINITIONS
Primary Colors
Red, Yellow, Blue
Secondary Colors
Mixture of two Primary Colors.
Intermediate Colors
One Primary and one Secondary mixed together.
Complementary Mixed Colors
Mixed colors directly opposite each other.

Hue: Another name for color.
Tint: Color + White.
Tone: Color + Grey.
Shade: Color + Black.
Neutral Grey:
Mixture of 3 Primary Colors of Black + White.
Intensity or Chroma:
The brightness or dullness of a color.
Value:
The lightness or darkness of a color.

THE COLOR WHEEL

Know your color wheel! The benefit of knowing colors and how to combine them not only gives you a professional edge, but eliminates excessive cost in buying extra products for your kit. A complete understanding includes knowing how to create tints, tones, and shades using the art of blending and mixing colors.

All colors begin from mixing primary colors, which are red, yellow, and blue. When a cosmetic company creates a color, the chemist will use the same methods of mixing and blending that an artist would use, adding pearl to create shimmer. Powders, liquids, creams, and other formulations create the variety of products that are available to the consumer.

THE LANGUAGE OF COLOR

Primary colors: Red, yellow, and blue

Secondary colors: The mixture of two primary colors. Example:

   mixing red and yellow = orange

   red and blue = violet

   yellow and blue = green

Intermediate colors: Combine one primary and one secondary color. Example:

   red and orange = red-orange

   blue and green = blue-green

Most eyeshadow colors are combinations of intermediate colors.

Complementary colors: Colors directly opposite each other on the color wheel. When two complementary colors are placed next to each other, they enhance or brighten each other. In terms of makeup application, if you use a reddish violet hue on a green eye or an orange or rust hue on a blue eye, the effect will be to enhance the eye color. Since complementary colors neutralize when mixed, using a yellow-based concealer on a bluish-purple undereye discoloration minimizes the effect. A green tinted foundation or base neutralizes ruddy tones in the skin.

Tint: Any color mixed with white.

Tone: Any color mixed with grey.

Shade: Color plus black.

You can acquire a wide spectrum of colors by adding tints, tones, or shades to primary and secondary colors.

Intensity or **chroma:** A term that refers to the brightness or dullness of a color.

Value: Refers to a color's lightness or darkness. For example, mixing black eyeshadow and white, depending on the proportion of each color, will result in a whole spectrum of greys.

In general, shading is for contouring, and tinting is for highlighting.

Hue: Another name for color.

Monochromatic hue: Refers to a color with various values of black, white, and grey. For example, if you mix blue with white, the result is pale blue. If you add black to blue, the result is teal blue.

Achromatic hue: Refers to a colorless scheme of black, white, and grey.

lighting

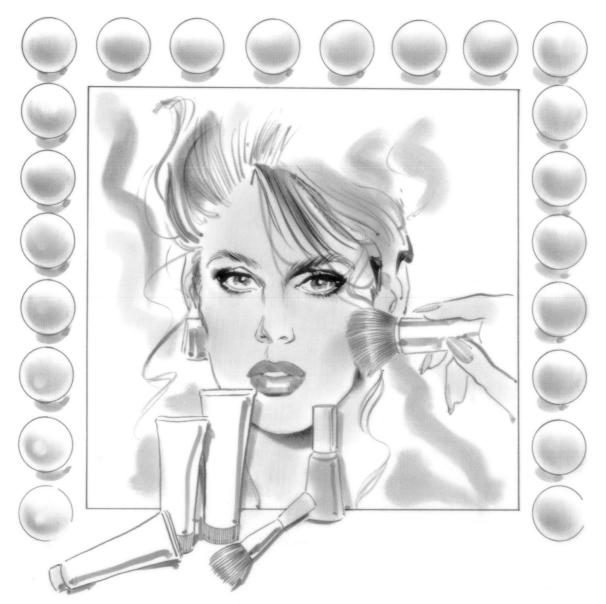

The lighting source must be correct to ensure the best possible results when applying makeup to the face. Many consumers are often misled by judging the cosmetic products they purchase under the incorrect lighting source. It is important to practice the guidelines below prior to applying makeup to the face. Using the correct light source can eliminate many problems, including wrong color selection and shadows on the face. The setup of your working area can vary; I use two types of setups for both my studio and on-location work. Whether you are applying your makeup at home or setting up a workstation at your place of business, I recommend the following setup. Some makeup mirrors sold in retail stores resemble professional makeup mirrors; unfortunately these mirrors are too small for professional use.

Surrounding the top and sides of the mirror, a lighting source should be available. The best possible lighting arrangement is one that allows you to apply makeup based on the light you or your client will be under. For example, if someone is to be made up for an occasion that will be held outdoors in natural light, you would not apply makeup that is suited for soft pink or diffused lighting. This is why it is important to be aware of the colors that different light sources emit and how to determine your application procedure accordingly. If a natural light source is available, set up your mirror approximately six to eight feet from the natural light source and let the light reflect toward the face; natural lighting is best for outdoor daytime makeup or special outdoor occasions. A selection of both incandescent (most flattering) and fluorescent (least flattering) bulbs should be installed into a strip light surrounding the mirror. An alternating mix of blue, green, red, and yellow lights is the ultimate lighting source, so you can adjust the lights according to the lighting situation and the client's needs.

I recommend using a diffused or frosted bulb to avoid excess glare on the mirror. In addition to the mirror setup, avoid bright or dark walls; surround the area with neutral walls or softly patterned neutral wallcoverings. A pale grey or neutral buff shade is best.

FLUORESCENT LIGHTING

Fluorescent light is used in many office buildings and places of business and consists mainly of unflattering blue and green rays, which can create a harsh and unhealthy skintone in the face. Due to the undertones in fluorescent light, any blue undertones on the facial skin are overenhanced and must be corrected; for example, an undereye discoloration is usually more pronounced in a fluorescent lighting situation and must be corrected using a yellow-beige concealer if there are violet undertones beneath the skin. If white or light beige was applied, the area would appear ashy and artificial looking. The best color palette to use contains softer shades of pinks or hues in the blue/red family. Selecting this color palette will help avoid a drab, washed-out, unhealthy look in the face. Avoid heavy application of dark, overpowering colors, and keep makeup as sheer as possible, making sure to correct any discolorations or blemishes on the face.

In fluorescent light, avoid:

❏ Heavy frosted or pearlized highlighters anywhere on the face.

❏ Deep, dark eyeliners around the eyes or lips or any harsh, overenhanced features.

❏ Too much yellow base or foundation. This is the only lighting for which I recommend using a tint of red or pink to avoid a muddy look in the skin. (Use concealer only to remove violet undertones; follow with a tinted foundation.)

❏ Ash brown or warm beige shades. If a natural look is desired, opt for reddish-browns or cool beiges that will not appear drab on the face.

❏ Heavy application of any products to the face; try to keep skin moist and hydrated looking, yet not too shiny or powdery looking.

INCANDESCENT LIGHTING

Incandescent lighting emits red and yellow rays and is the most flattering of all light sources. Usually this type of lighting is used in restaurants, catering halls, and theaters. Although it is an artificial light source, it is the makeup artist's most favored light source. Unlike with fluorescent light, a makeup artist can create a warmer skintone using beige or golden undertones and can also use a heavier base application, allowing for more coverage to perfect the skin.

Professional Tip: Keep the foundation a half a shade paler to lighten and brighten the skintone. Use pearls or high-lighters to lift and enhance features, and a color palette of your choice can be used. As always, when applying makeup I recommend blending well to create an attractive look no matter what amount of product you are using. Many people make the mistake of "overdoing" themselves or others for special occasions. The ability to enhance the face no matter what the lighting source is the sign of a good makeup application.

LIGHTING TIPS

❏ Light should fall on the face from around the sides and top of the mirror to allow an even distribution of rays.

❏ Never allow light to fall directly from above or below the face; this will cast too many shadows on the face.

❏ A strip light with alternating incandescent and fluorescent lights is best suited for most applications. Daylight is a combination of red, yellow, blue, and green rays. Therefore, for daylight you can use all the lights; for evening or warm lighting use the incandescent lights; and for office lighting use the fluorescent lights.

❏ Lighting strips are available at many hardware stores and lighting centers and are relatively inexpensive.

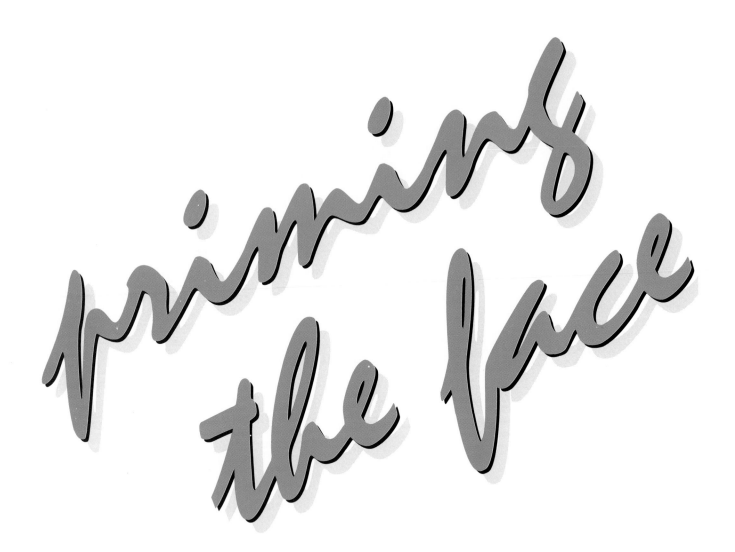

priming the face

concealing techniques

DAVID HAMSLEY

Proper use of concealers is one of the most important subjects a makeup artist should master. This aspect of makeup application helps to correct discolorations and/or highlight recessed areas on the face. Before choosing a concealer, you must decide whether the concealer will be used for (a) correcting discoloration (b) highlighting recessed areas or (c) both. Depending on its use, you will then be able to choose the proper concealer, color, and coverage.

TEXTURE

Concealers are manufactured in many consistencies, including cream pots, pencils, sticks, tubes, and powder-cream bases. Whichever product you choose, a thorough understanding of how to use the product is extremely important in order to achieve the most effective results.

Cream pot: Usually known to have a high color pigment (very good coverage) and when applied is easy to control. Look for a pot concealer that has a low oil content, that is tacky to the touch, and that blends smoothly.

Sticks: Sold in a lipstick tube case, this formulation is common on the retail market, is usually very heavy on the delicate skin under the eyes, is easy to carry, and is convenient for on-the-spot touch-ups.

Pencils: Depending on the formulation, concealer pencils are rarely sold in retail stores. However, several professional makeup companies formulate jumbo pencils that are compact, offer excellent coverage, and are easy to use.

Tubes: Squeeze and wand type containers are usually formulated with a higher oil content to create a liquid consistency, which is best if used for highlighting features, not as a color corrector.

Powder-cream: If applied too heavily, this formulation can appear lined and caked under a foundation. It is great for taut skin that needs minimal coverage. Works best accompanied by a matte powder base for black and white photography makeup.

My favorite consistency is the cream pot concealer, which is tacky to the touch, easy to blend, and in my opinion offers the most effective and natural looking coverage.

When choosing a concealer look for a formulation that offers an easy-to-mix (custom blend) formula, low oil content, and highly pigmented base.

COLOR

Color choice is another priority when using concealing techniques. When selecting a concealer keep in mind that the product will be applied to correct discolorations or to highlight recessed areas on the face. For both situations, the color you choose depends entirely on the area to be corrected. One of the most common mistakes many people make is misunderstanding when to use a corrective shade and when to use a highlighting shade.

Corrective concealer is used to minimize dark or discolored skin under and around the eyes, at the corners of nostrils, and on any facial blemishes.

The most prevalent color in undereye discoloration is usually a pale purple or eggplant color. To neutralize this color, I use the opposite shade on the color wheel, which is a maize (corn yellow) or mustard shade. I would custom mix a pale or deep beige cream concealer with a yellow cream. I recommend mixing a shade that is closest to the depth of the skintone, then applying the product directly to the discoloration using a flat-edged tapered brush (see illustration).

For blemishes or ruddy (red) discolorations, an ash tone beige concealer will help to reduce redness. On blemishes, a second coat of concealer may be neccesary to apply after the foundation and prior to powdering the face. (Note: Depending on the severity of the discoloration, an application of foundation correctly applied can often achieve most of the coverage needed.)

When correcting a discolored area, apply the product directly to the area and use a minimum amount of product. Feather the edges, leave on the skin, and do not wipe or blend away. Less is more! You will discover why this step is important when we learn about foundations.

Highlighting shades are used to "lift out" recessed or lined areas of the face. When depth is prevalent under the eyes and discoloration is not the problem, choose a beige tone concealer that is one or two shades lighter than the foundation to be applied.

This technique also works well to highlight deep facial lines and recessed facial areas. Simply apply the concealer to a fine sable liner brush and paint directly into the lined or recessed area. (Note: Blend the edges and do not blend outside of the line.)

Puffiness beneath the eyes must be corrected using a different technique. Apply a highlighting shade to a fine liner brush; then apply the liner to the edge of the entire recessed area surrounding the puff. Apply the selected shade of foundation to the face, taking caution not to "blend away" the highlight. Next mix a foundation one-and-a-half to two shades darker and apply directly to the puff. You will notice how this special technique creates the illusion of a less prominent puff.

To conceal scars use the techniques described above. If the skin has a protruding or recessed scar, this is considered three dimensional. The professional makeup techniques described in this section will help you to achieve the illusion of less prominence. I recommend never making the false claim that you can remove a scar with makeup; however, with practice you will be able to conceal with unbelievable results.

SPECIAL NOTES

Never pull or stretch the area beneath the eyes, since this area of facial skin is very delicate and special care should be taken when applying these products.

Application techniques for all of the above products should be as follows: Use a warming process by applying each product to a flat sable brush, then mixing on the top of the hand to bring to body temperature, gently apply to the area to be concealed or highlighted.

foundation

Foundation to a makeup artist is as important as canvas to an artist. When an artist begins to paint a picture, the artist will usually use a primer coat to prepare for an even texture to the canvas. When applying makeup we will use an analogy to an artist; however the "canvas" will be the skin. Foundation applied correctly can help accomplish several things: coverage, color, protection, and a radiant glow or perfect finish to the skin.

Several variables must be considered prior to selecting foundation for the skin you will be working on.

SKIN TEXTURE

Before selecting foundation the skin's texture must be analyzed. Does the skin have large pores (similar to an orange peel), tight pores (an apple), three-dimensional indentations or protrusions (a deep scar, moles, or blemishes)? One important rule in professional makeup is to remember that you are not a surgeon, and although you can help diminish three-dimensional skin problems you can never remove them, but can only give the illusion of less prominence using the corrective application techniques described in this section.

SKINTONE

The color of the skin is a very important factor to consider prior to makeup application. My experience with many of the retail lines available on today's market is that there are too many peach or pink pigments in the product. Realistically most people do not have this skintone, so it is not a good color choice. When analyzing skin, you can categorize four tones:

    normal — a natural, healthy looking color

    sallow — a yellowish-blue undertone

    olive — a greenish cast to the skin

    ruddy — a reddish color to the skin

When choosing a foundation, I often refer to a color scale that goes from ivory to ebony, working with natural beige or yellow tones rather than peach or pink. I feel that a make-up artist should never try to simulate a natural looking skintone with these shades.

Although you can add a hint of red or bronze to the foundation to add a glow of color, this should be mixed into the foundation and spot applied rather than applied to the entire face (common for a natural looking male makeup application). I recommend never choosing a product simply by the color name. For example, thousands of shades are labeled ivory or natural beige, and they probably range from peach or pink to true beige tones. (Always test the product for color, coverage, and consistency.)

SKIN TYPE

Depending on the skin type, the formulation of foundation you choose is very important. For oily skin choose a foundation that has low or no oil content; for dry skin opt for a moisture-based foundation; and for normal skin a foundation for normal skin types is recommended.

THE THREE C'S
Color

When testing a foundation, color choice is a very important factor. The color you choose must match the skin exactly to assure the most natural results. When choosing a shade to match the skin, I recommend testing it beneath the jawline and the ear. Choose a shade that best matches the natural skintone and apply to the area.

Oxidation may occur if the foundation is not warmed to body temperature prior to applying the makeup base. Through experience I have discovered that any cream makeup applied at room temperature must first be warmed to test the true color and consistency on the face. An example would be if you were to apply a cream foundation base when the room temperature is 60 degrees. If you were to apply the product directly to the face, more product than is actually needed would be applied. The face will then warm the product to body temperature, causing it to oxidize, and a color change will occur.

Always warm any cream products to body temperature before testing or applying to the face. This technique is simple and results in clean, perfect color and a perfect amount of coverage. To apply this method, simply use the top part of the hand between the thumb and pointer finger as a palette. Apply a small amount of product, wait a moment, and see the results for yourself. It's amazing how accurately this method works when applying cream products. Let the product warm and change color on your hand; then, using a wedge, apply to the face.

Consistency

The formulation you choose depends on the consistency of the product. Foundations come in several consistencies ranging from water based, which offers the lightest coverage, to moisture based, which offers a bit more coverage combined with moisturizing ingredients, to cream based, which is heaviest in consistency and oil content.

Coverage

Depending on the type of makeup application and skin condition, foundation coverage varies. If the skin is naturally flawless (free of discolorations or blemishes), you can usually use a light, water-based foundation to even the skintone. For skin with minimal discolorations, a slightly heavier foundation that offers natural coverage should be fine. And for skin that needs heavier coverage or to achieve a flawless look, a cream-based foundation would be your best choice.

When applying foundation, use a moistened latex wedge that simulates natural skin pores to apply the makeup base. It is important that you never use the fingertips to apply foundation; not only is this unsanitary, the excess product is left on the skin, and the oils on the fingers can cause a discoloration on the face. When applying foundation, use the warming process described above; then lightly apply the product starting at the forehead and blending downward toward the jawline. Never rub hard on the face or pull the skin while applying the base. I often refer to the frosting a cake analogy. Imagine frosting a chocolate cake with white frosting. In order to achieve a perfect looking cake, you will need to apply the white very carefully to ensure even coverage.

After applying the foundation, use a water-moistened clean wedge to remove excess coverage and to achieve a natural finish to the makeup before powdering the face. This is called hydrating the base. The areas that will need to be moistened are the deep nasolabial folds (laugh lines), any lines around the eyes, and any areas that do not need excess coverage. (*Note*: For aging skin with deep lines or a wrinkled appearance, it is best to use a lighter formulation; a heavy cream makeup will tend to look unnatural.)

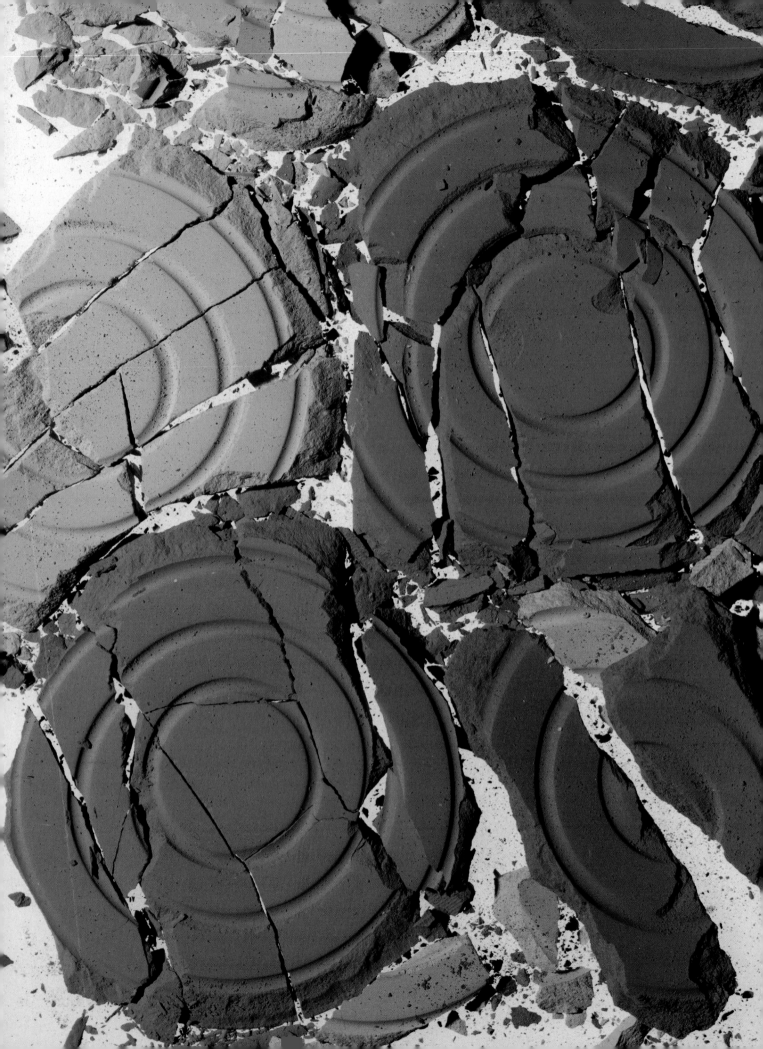

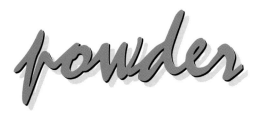

Puff it on, press it on, buff it on. Whichever way you apply it, powder was originally designed to absorb excess oils, add color, and reduce shine on the face. With today's advanced technology, however, powder has been designed to do much more than that!

Powder can be used to tint, tone, and highlight the face according to the shade you select. Prior to selecting a powder, there are several qualities to look for.

1. **Coverage:** How does the product color and adhere to the skin? A good quality powder should offer even color distribution and should adhere to the face.

2. **Slip:** How does the powder feel? Roll the powder between your fingers; it should feel like silk. Soft and fine — never grainy. The finer milled the powder is, the finer the application.

3. **Absorbency:** How does the powder absorb oils and excess shine? A fine quality powder will not appear cakey or "break the oil barrier" in a minimal amount of time. (*Tip*: To remove powder from lines or crevices, press a water-moistened cotton pad over the area and roll off. Never wipe or press too hard. This will lift off the caked area.)

I opt for a transparent, "no color" loose powder for most applications. This choice of neutral powder does not change the color, yet absorbs excess shine on the face.

Translucent powders are tinted with color and are available in a variety of shades. For deeper skintones, choose a golden ochre or deeper yellow shade; for paler skins, a natural beige or neutral shade.

Use colored powders to tint or tone down the shade of the face. Violet can be used to lift a sallow or yellow skintone. Mint can be used to tone down ruddiness or red skintones. Peach can help add a glow to the skin, and white is an excellent highlighting shade.

Powders are available in both pressed compact and loose forms. I recommend using both. Loose powders can be applied using a velour puff — simply shake a little powder onto the puff, then fold together to distribute the color. Next press and roll the powder over the face. Avoid pulling or rubbing onto the face; this will result in a smeared makeup application. Buff the excess powder using a sable brush. Pressed powders are convenient for touch-ups and can be pressed or buffed onto the face. Bronzing powders and highlighting or shimmer powders are usually available in pressed powder form. For evening or special occasion makeup, you can add shimmer to the shoulders, cleavage, or back simply by using any of the above powders.

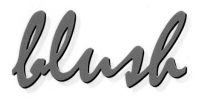

Blush is used to add definition, accentuate the cheekbones, and add the finishing touch to the foundation of the face. Blush is the one step that really makes a difference in the makeup application.

Blush brings back or restores the "healthy glow" to a skintone that is lacking color balance or a face that has been primed with foundation. In addition to adding color, blush can help accentuate facial features and, applied properly, can change the appearance of the facial structure.

APPLICATION

The guideline that is most accurate to follow when applying blush is to locate the outer pupil of the eye (toward the ear) and the bottom bridge of the nose (beneath the nostrils). If you create an imaginary line, vertically down the cheek from the outer pupil, then horizontally from the base of the nose toward the ear, you would locate the notch of the ear. This area is where the cheekbone is located. Blush should always be put on starting from the outer part of the face going toward the center. If you begin your blush at the front of the cheek, you deposit the largest portion of color in front of the face, which can create the illusion of a fuller or blotchy cheek. Think of a hollow tunnel; the darkest area is the bottom. A cheekbone should naturally have more depth toward the back of the face, then gradually come toward the front of the face.

Depending on the bone structure, blush can be applied to help enhance or distract from facial features.

❏ A long or narrow face can appear to have more width simply by applying color horizontally at the cheekbone.

❏ A short or round face can be lengthened by applying blush in a triangular pattern blended upward toward the temples.

❏ A square-shaped face can be softened by applying a circular pattern at the cheek area (using the main guideline) toward the ear and accenting the circular pattern at the fullest area of the cheek.

❏ Attractive eyes can be accentuated by adding a splash of color at the brows; lips can be enhanced with a hint of color at the chin.

Choosing a color scheme for blush depends on the color palette that you are working with in your makeup application. I recommend choosing a color that is not dominantly in the warm or cool color scheme. If you choose a palette of natural peach shadow, warm cinnamon lipstick, and soft brown liner, choose a blush in the warm peach or reddish brown family. For a cool palette, mauve shadows and pink lip shades would look best with a cooler shade of cheek color.

My personal preference is a powder-type
blush formula for most of my makeup applications. Powders are easy to blend, especially
when you are trying to alter and mix with
other colors. For severely lined or dehydrated
skin, I will usually use a cream or gel formula
to add a moist, healthy look to the skin.
Before applying blush, you must first determine what formula you will choose.

Powders or powder-cream formulas are
applied using a blush brush. I recommend a
brush with natural pony or sable hair; syn-
thetics can be abrasive to the skin. Powdered
blush must be applied after powdering or setting the face with a powder. If a colored blush
is applied to moist skin, the color pigments will
"grab" the moisture and a blotchy skintone
will develop. When applying blush, dip the
brush lightly into the color, then tap excess
color onto a tissue and apply to the cheek or to
any areas where blush is needed. If a line of
demarcation occurs, or the shade selected has
too much color value depth, simply dip the
brush into loose, transparent powder; then
blend it with the desired color and apply to
the cheek.

Gel or cream formulas should be applied to a
face that has been prepared with a moisturizer
and a foundation. The cream will allow the
product to blend smoothly onto the face. You

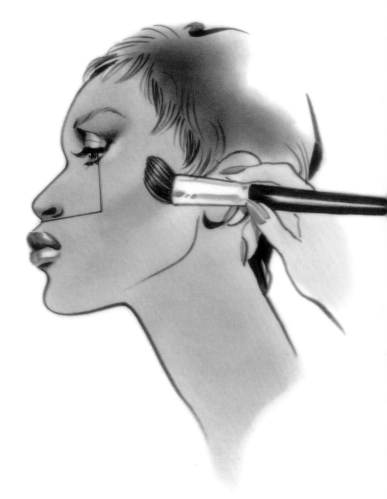

can use a wedge or sponge to apply the color,
being careful to apply a minimum amount of
pigment and adding more if necessary. This formula must be applied prior to setting the makeup with any type of powder and should not be
applied after powdering the face.

The goal of using blush is to give the illusion of
health to the face. It should be soft, natural,
and understated unless otherwise intended.
Always powder any blush applied to the face
and blend away any harsh lines of demarcation.

eyes

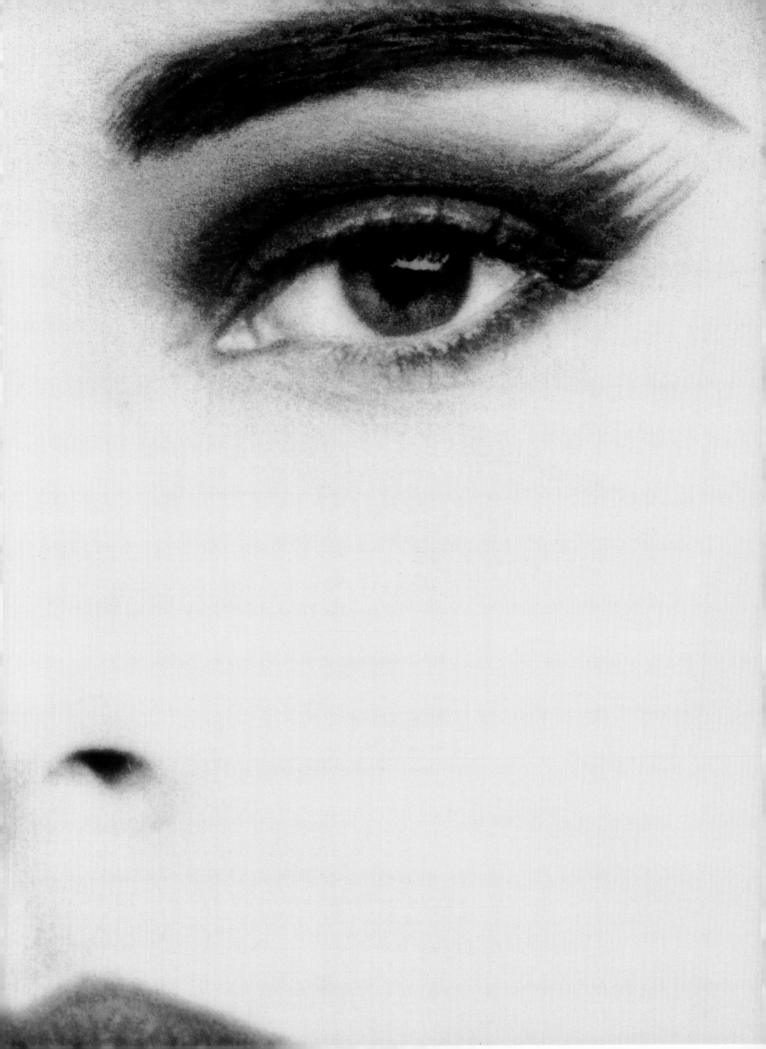

eyebrows

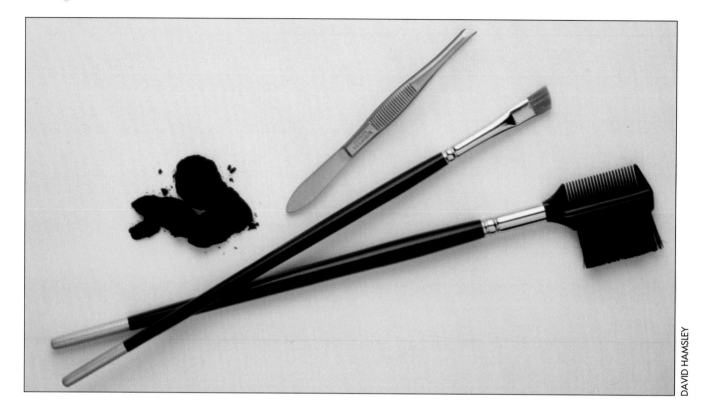

Eyebrows are the frame to a beautiful picture, the eyes. Properly groomed and shaped brows help enhance and add expression to the face and are without doubt an essential step to completing any makeup application.

With or without makeup, grooming the eyebrows should be a part of your daily routine. Prior to grooming, shaping, or coloring the brows, refer to the following guidelines in order to achieve the best possible results.

TOOLS

Tweezers

There are several styles of tweezers to choose from: square, round, pointed, and slant-tipped. I prefer a precision-made slant-tip tweezer; the angular tip is easiest to control. When using a tweezer always remove hair in the direction it grows from the follicle; apply an astringent to follow.

Depilatory Wax

Waxing can be used to remove an abundance of hair beneath the arch or in the center of the brows. I personally do not recommend using the waxing method to achieve a complete brow shaping; however, removing excess hair with wax, then completing the shaping with a tweezer is fine. Most people will only require tweezer shaping.

Brow Brush/Comb

This is a dual-sided tool used to brush and comb the brow hairs into shape.

BROW MAKEUP

Brow Set or Gel

This is a clear liquid gel available in a mascara tube, formulated to dry matte and hold brow hairs in place. (Do not confuse this product with colorless mascara, which can result in a shiny appearance.)

Eyebrow Pencils

Pencils are available in a variety of shades and formulations. I recommend using a pencil to fill in the brows, followed by an application of powdered shadow to set and soften the brow.

Powdered Eyeshadow

Apply natural matte shades using a stiff, angular shadow brush to create a soft, natural look.

HOW TO SHAPE THE BROWS

When shaping the brows, it is important to use a guideline to ensure an even looking shape. Usually the natural shape of the upper lid matches the natural arch of the eyebrow. The brow should start above the inner corner of the eye and end at the outer corner of the eye toward the temple area. You can measure this by using the end of the brow comb handle and holding it at a diagonal from the bottom of the nostril to the outer edge of the eye. This will be the guideline for eyeshadows.

Eyeshadow should not exend beyond this point unless intended. The natural shape of the brow is fuller at the inner corner and tapers toward the outer ends.

Most brows will have excess hair at the center of the eyes and beneath the natural arch. It is important to remove the excess hair carefully using a slanted tweezer and removing hair in the direction of the hair growth. If the eyes are very closely set, you may want to remove the hair slightly beyond the inner corner of the brow to help achieve the illusion that the eyes are further apart. The same technique applies for wide-set eyes; you can bring the brows closer to the center of the eyes using a brow pencil or shadow to give the illusion of natural hair. I recommend using a brow brush after filling in the brows to create the look of natural hair growth.

When choosing the correct color for the brows, apply a shade that is a step lighter than the natural hair color. If the situation calls for an overpowered eyebrow (i.e., a high, arched, dramatic brow), you would use a deeper shade of brown or black/brown to achieve this look. If the natural brow hair is too dark for the face, you can lighten it professionally, with a hair tint, or a lighter powder.

Some eyebrows tend to grow out of shape and can create an odd look to the face. In these cases you should use corrective brow shaping techniques. Follow the guide below for special situations that need extra attention.

Bushy Brows

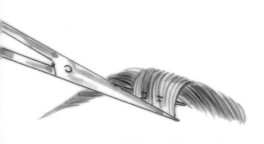

Using a brow brush, brush the hairs downward toward the eyelid; then, using a small scissor, trim the excess hair, following the shape of the natural arch of the brow. Then comb into shape.

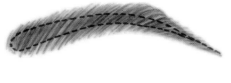

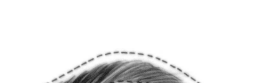

Thin Brows

Draw a guideline that matches both brows; then fill in the brows with the desired color and brush to create natural-looking hair strokes.

High-arched Brows

Remove hair from the upper arch of the brow to create length; then fill in the excess hair beneath the arch to give a lengthier appearance.

Sparse Brows

Measure the eyes using the guideline below; make a dot where the brow should begin and end; then fill in to desired thickness and shape with either a brow pencil or shadow.

Note: Depending on a person's face shape (long, round, square, or oval), changing the shape of the brows can help to achieve balance in the face and alter the appearance. For example, if a person's face is very square, you may want to add an arch at the center to add length to the face, therefore eliminating the square look.

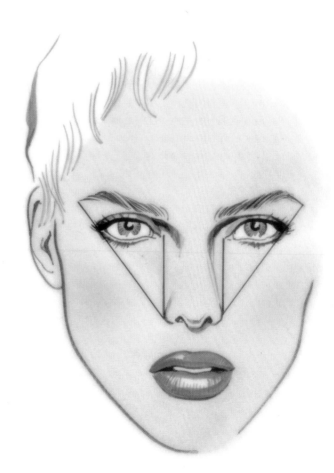

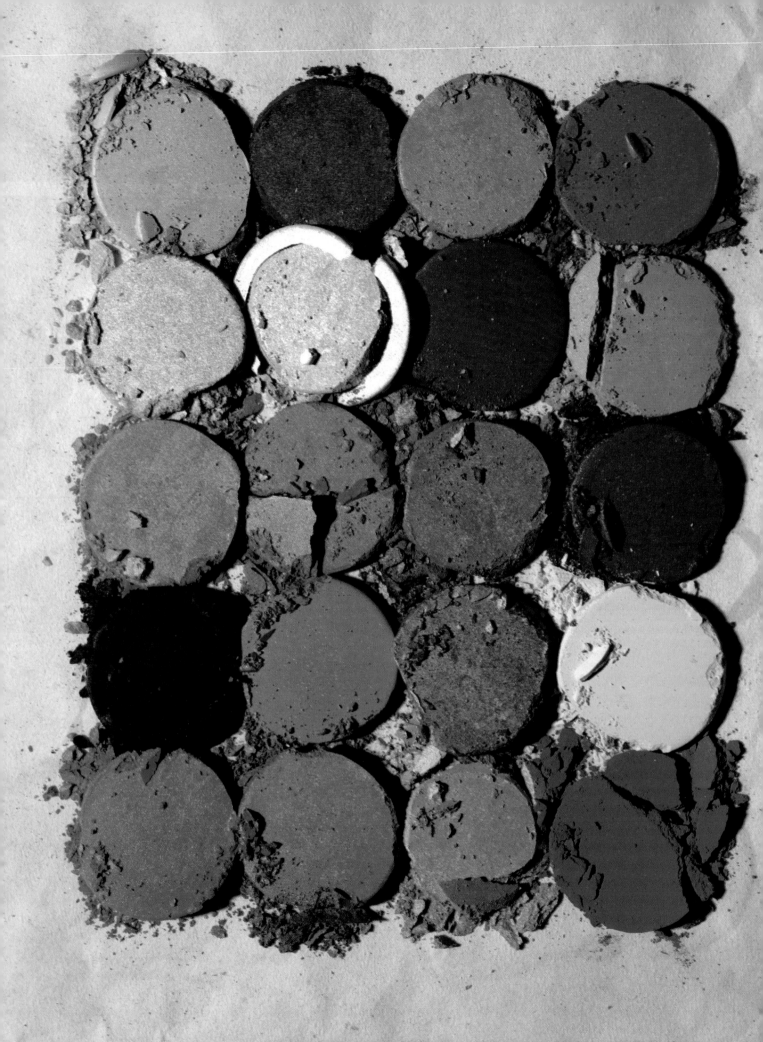

eyeshadow

Dramatic, soft, shimmery, smoky, or natural eyes can all be achieved by expertly chosen color and careful placement of eyeshadow. Eyeshadow, when applied properly, can bring focus to one of the most important features of the face. Applying eyeshadow is more than merely sweeping any color over the lid to finish the look. Although some eyes can handle a sweep of color, most eyes need a little extra help to reshape, contour, highlight, or define the feature.

Before applying eyeshadow, make sure you have the following tools available.

Brushes:

❏ **Tight, angular shadow brush** — for definition around the base of the lids.

❏ **Small fluff shadow brush** — for application of shadow to the base of the eyelids.

❏ **Large, chiseled fluff brush** — for contouring shadow into the crease of the eye and blending the shadows.

❏ **Sponge eyeshadow applicators** — if desired. I personally find that it is difficult to control the amount of product when using these applicators, resulting in an uneven application. Because of this, I do not recommend their use.

Other items:

❏ **Small tissue** — folded into a wedge shape. Use to place beneath the eyes when applying shadows to the lid (catches excess powder, which can cause discoloration under the eyes).

❏ **Latex wedge** — to blend shadows at the outer corners of the eye.

❏ **Cotton swabs** — to lift off unwanted shadow.

❏ **Small water dish** — to apply the shadows wet.

❏ **Lid primer or foundation and powder** — as a shadow base.

APPLICATION TECHNIQUES

When applying eyeshadow, it is important to analyze the consistency of the shadow product you will be working with. Several formulations of shadows are available; therefore it is important to test a few products to see what type of product you prefer. Cream eyeshadow is usually very thick and the color pigment is concentrated, making it difficult to apply and blend. Cream shadows are not commonly used in professional makeup because of this inconvenience. The most commonly used shadows are the pressed powder type, which offer a variety of mattes, pearls, and demi-pearls and the convenience of color control depending on the amount applied. Powdered shadows are also easy to blend, and most of the powders can be applied wet or dry.

It is important to feel the shadow and test the texture prior to using the product. I prefer using a creamy powdered shadow (not too dry). Powder types adhere to the skin and result in minimal or no flaking.

When applying eyeshadow, choose your color palette and apply according to the eye shape you are working on. Keep in mind that light, bright, or pearlized shades will highlight or bring out areas, and dark, dull, or matte shades recede the eye.

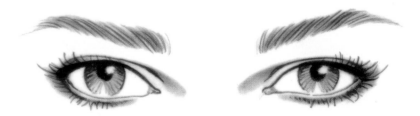

Close-set Eyes

Apply a lighter shade of color to the inner corners. This will give the illusion of width to the eye. Then extend the outer corners of the eyes by using darker shades of color and blending well to bring attention to the outer corners. Remove the brow hairs beyond the inner corner of the eye and apply eyeliner starting at the center of the base of the lid and extending to the outer corners of the eye.

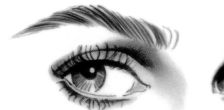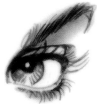

Deep-set Eyes

Use a light, reflective color on the eyelids to lift out the eyes. Then apply a contour shade above the crease of the eye and blend outward to give the illusion of a bone. Highlight above the contour shade and apply mascara to lift the eyes and blend all shadows well.

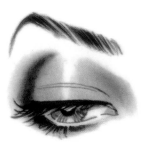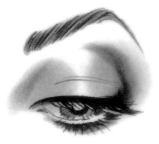

Protruding Eyes

Apply dark, dull, or matte shades over the entire lid, extending the color above the crease of the eye. Add a highlight color to the area beneath the arch of the brow bone, and blend well. Apply eyeliner to the base of the upper and lower lids. Apply mascara toward the base of the lashes and avoid light or bright colors on the lids. You may also want to rim the inner eyelid with a deeper shade of liner to further recede the eye.

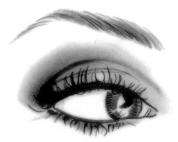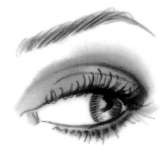

Wide-set Eyes

Apply a darker shade of color at the inner corner of the eye near the bridge of the nose. Then apply lighter shades toward the outer part of the eye. Extend brows toward the bridge of the nose and apply an extra coat of mascara to the inner lashes of the eye.

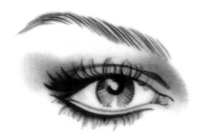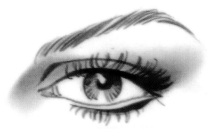

Drooping Eyes

Create the illusion of lifted eyes by applying eyeliner starting at the inner corners of the lid and extending outward toward the outer center of the upper lid. Then extend the liner just above the natural line of the lid to "lift" the line upward. Apply a deeper contour shadow above the liner and sweep upward and outward at the outer corner of the eye. Apply a lighter shadow at the inner crease and above the brow bone. Use a liner at the lower lash area and extend outward and upward at the outer corners. Finish the eyes by applying mascara almost to the end of the natural lashes, creating an upward lift.

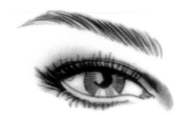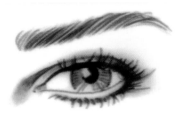

Small Eyes

Use lighter, brighter, and paler shades on the lids to open the eyes. Add a shading color at the outer edge of the crease to lengthen the eyelids. Apply a generous application of mascara to the end of the lashes.

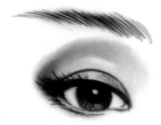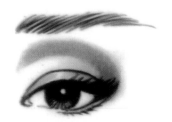

Almond-shaped Eyes

Create the illusion of a crease by applying a pale shade at the inner third of the eye, positioned vertically. Then apply a crease shade by contouring at the outer half of the lid. Add a strip of natural looking artificial lashes to lengthen lash hair.

eyeliner

Eyeliners add definition to the eyes and are a key item in your makeup collection. Liners can be used to elongate and lift the outer corners of the eyes, enhance or alter eyeshapes, and come in a variety of textures and formulations. They can also be used to add color to both the inner rim and the outer eyelid.

One of the questions I hear most often is "How can I keep my eyeliner from smearing or wearing off?" Depending on the product you use, there are ways to avoid this common problem.

Listed below are several types of eyeliners available on the market and application techniques for each.

CAKE EYELINER

This formulation, the choice of most professionals, is sold in a small shadow pan and should be applied using a fine eyeliner brush dipped into the moistened cake liner. Depending on the depth of color you desire, add more droplets for a lighter, thinner consistency or fewer droplets for a thicker consistency. I personally favor cake eyeliner because I can control the lines and color to achieve the results I desire. I also like the effect of using fresh water to apply the product, which is that it creates a smooth matte finish on the lid.

LIQUID EYELINER

This formulation, premade and packaged in a tube, is drying to the delicate skin around the eyes and tends to dry shiny, to crack, and to flake. In addition, you have no control over the color or consistency of the product, and it is usually packaged with an inexpensive synthetic brush.

PENCIL EYELINERS

Pencil eyeliners are made in a variety of formulations and sizes ranging from thin to jumbo. They usually have a waxy consistency (helps to keep the form and makes them easy to apply). Pencils come in the widest variety of colors and are easy to smudge and blend. A problem with pencils is that they tend to wear off or smear when left on the skin. To combat this problem, select a matching powdered eyeshadow and apply using a tapered angular shadow brush directly over the pencil to set. Pencil eyeliners are the choice for coloring the inner base of the eyelids.

EYELINER PENS

Eyeliner pens are similar to liquid eyeliner and have a pointed felt-tip or brush applicator, similar to a marker pen. They are easy to use and work well for quick, easy applications. Again, the control of color is not available, and for professional use they are unsanitary because the applicator is built into the pen.

When using eyeliner, control the amount of liner by tapering the color at the base of the lids. Never apply one thick or thin stroke of color along the entire lashline (unless intended). It can tend to look too harsh. Liner should be applied based on the shape and size of the eye (see illustrations of eye shapes on pages 62 – 64).

mascara

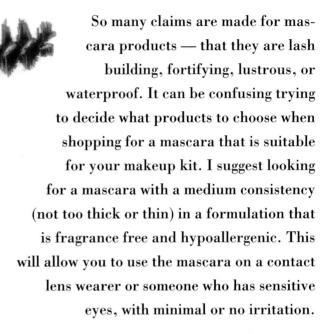

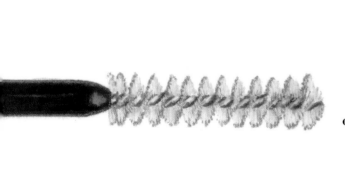

So many claims are made for mascara products — that they are lash building, fortifying, lustrous, or waterproof. It can be confusing trying to decide what products to choose when shopping for a mascara that is suitable for your makeup kit. I suggest looking for a mascara with a medium consistency (not too thick or thin) in a formulation that is fragrance free and hypoallergenic. This will allow you to use the mascara on a contact lens wearer or someone who has sensitive eyes, with minimal or no irritation.

I use two mascara formulations in my professional makeup kit: original formula and water-resistant mascara. Original formula is used for most makeup applications requiring a basic coverage to enhance and color the lashes. This formula is water soluble and easy to remove. Water-resistant mascara is used for waterproof makeup, for special occasions requiring tearproof makeup, and for hot and humid days when the skin is moist or perspiring.

Water-resistant mascara is usually very drying to the delicate lash hairs. When removing this product use a quality eye makeup remover applied to a cotton square and gently remove the product, sweeping downward with the lid closed, then inward under the eyes toward the bridge of the nose. Repeat until the lashes are clean.

COLOR CHOICE

Use the following guidelines when choosing a mascara color.

❏ Pale blondes and redheads: soft brown or sable.

❏ Light or medium brunettes to black hair: black or black brown.

❏ An attention-getting shade for most eyes: black.

❏ Mascara is also available in a variety of shades. Although I rarely use colored mascara, the following shades can also be used to enhance the lashes: a selection of blues, browns, greens, greys, and plums.

APPLICATION TECHNIQUE

Prior to applying mascara, unless the lashes are naturally curled, I recommend using an eyelash curler on the upper lashes. Not only does this help to open the eye, it also "fans" the lash hairs so they appear more evenly distributed on the lid base.

Using the Lash Curler

Carefully place the edge of the rubber base of the lash curler on the upper lashes so that the lashes are on the base; keep rubber away from the skin of the eyelid. Next, depending on the amount of curl desired, press the curler, gently adding slight pressure to the handle. I usually use one to three firm pressings, depending on the results I want to achieve. Although some people use the curler after applying mascara, I do not recommend doing this. It can cause the mascara to clump and flake, and it can grab and pull out lash hairs.

Applying Mascara

Using the mascara of your choice, dip the wand into the base of the container and fill the wand with the color. Next dot the tip of the wand on a tissue to remove the excess mascara from the top of the applicator (this is an important step, and if not done can result in a clumpy, uneven distribution of product to the lashes).

Holding the wand in a vertical position, begin to apply the mascara from the tip of the wand horizontally (back and forth), working from the base of the lashes to the tip. Rest your pinky finger on the chin for balance, and distribute the color evenly on the upper lashes. Then turn the wand to a horizontal position and brush color through from the base of the lashes to the tips. This technique allows the color to coat each lash evenly, adding one to four coats depending on the thickness you desire. Let the mascara dry between each coat to eliminate clumping of the product.

I never use lash fillers (fiber-formulated mascara) because you cannot control the amount of fiber applied to the lashes. For extra thick lashes, I also recommend the following technique. Apply one to three coats of mascara. While the last coat is moist dust a light coating of fine powder onto the lashes. Then apply the final coat. As always, use an eyelash comb to separate the lashes.

When applying mascara to the lower lashes, keep the wand close to the base and apply a light coat of color to the lashes. Separate the lashes and keep this area soft and natural looking. I rarely apply mascara to the bottom lashes. For definition for the lower lashline, applying a natural looking liner to the base of the lash can create the look you need.

TRICK OF THE TRADE

Using the proper wand for applying mascara is important. I recommend carrying a selection of wands as special tools in your kit.

- ❏ **Curved brush** — Depending on length of lashes, this brush helps curl the lashes and evenly distribute the product. It is not recommended for lower lashes, since application can be difficult with this brush.

- ❏ **Duo-tapered or Christmas-tree-shaped spiral applicator** — This shape fills the brush with product and is great for building full-looking lashes (spiral shape creates good separation).

- ❏ **Single-tapered spiral brush** — Good for all lashes; delivers a moderate amount of product with very good separation qualities.

- ❏ **Short brush** — Ideal for bottom and corner lashes and hard-to-reach areas at the lash base.

In addition to a wand-type applicator, you can also use a mini-fan brush to add volume and color to the back of the upper lash base.

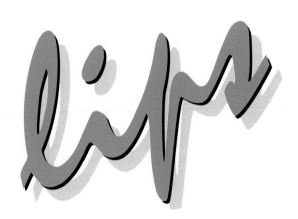

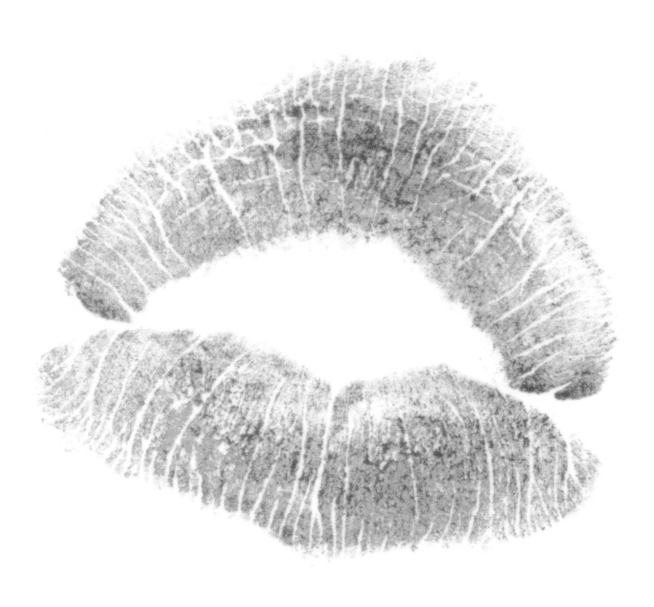

applying lip products

Matte, glossed, pale, or bold! Whatever look your makeup application calls for, well-applied and detailed lipcolor is a must for achieving professional-looking results. One of the most common mistakes is uneven application of lip products. The main reason this problem occurs is that the application techniques applied are incorrect. I recommend investing time in studying lipstick application. Plenty of practice using the corrector chart and a variety of application techniques and products will assure that you become a pro.

If necessary, I recommend removing any excess hair around the upper lip, using a depilatory cream or wax 24 hours prior to applying lipcolor. Excess hair will interfere with lip products and will result in an uneven or distracting appearance.

THE PRODUCTS

❏ **Tools:** Lip brush, cotton swab, single-ply tissues.

❏ **Lip balm:** Should be used daily as a healing and moisturizing base on the delicate lip area, which lacks oil glands. I recommend a soft balm that is colorless and not too shiny. I use a small, jar-type balm available at most pharmacies.

❏ **Concealer:** Natural beige tones for correcting lip shapes.

❏ **Lipliner pencils:** Are used to create definition and to reshape the lips. Liners are formulated using a concentrated amount of color and ingredients, therefore helping to create a longer lasting barrier for the lips. (For longer lasting lipcolor, simply shape and fill in the lips with a lipliner pencil.) (*Note*: When correcting lip shapes, use a lipliner that simulates the natural color of the lips. Nude and a soft, natural, reddish brown will cover most lip shades.)

❑ **Lipsticks:** Formulated in many textures and a variety of shades, the ideal lipstick stains the lips to the true color and will deliver staying power. Opt for a creamy texture, which will help add moisture to the lips. (**The tissue trick:** To achieve a matte finish, apply the cream lipcolor of your choice, then place a single-ply tissue over the lips. Next dust over the tissue with loose transparent powder and remove the tissue. Another layer of lipcolor can be applied and re-powdered to strengthen the color and to extend the staying power. Colored eyeshadow can also be used to add color and matte the lipstick. Simply apply the color to a cotton swab or applicator and press or roll over the lips.)

❑ **Lipgloss:** Available in a pot or tube, lipglosses are light reflective and create a shiny appearance for the lips. Available in pearls and creams, lipgloss can be used to highlight or to add a sheer finish to the lips.

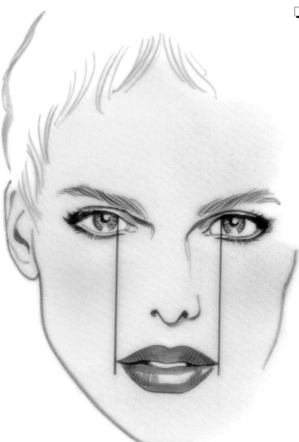

LIP CORRECTOR CHART

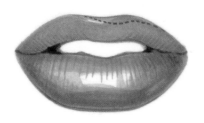

Uneven Lips

Create an even lip shape using a concealer and define with a tapered brush. Powder the lips; then apply lipliner to achieve the desired new lip shape, and fill with color.

Large or Full Lips

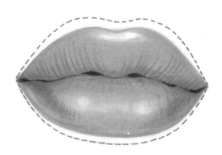

Apply a thin coat of foundation, then powder the lips. Selecting a deeper tone lipliner, line the inside of the natural lip and fill with a complimenting matte lip shade. (Avoid light, bright, or shiny colors.)

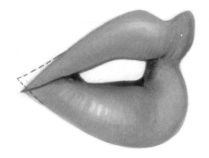

Drooping Lips

Lift the outer corners by applying concealer, then powdering the lips. Using the center line of the lips, draw a line upward at the outer corners, shape the lips, and fill with lipcolor.

Thin Lips

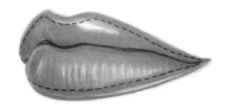

Using concealer, apply a thin line over the natural lipline and powder the lips. Next outline just above the natural lipline and fill with a light lipcolor or gloss. (Avoid dark or dull colors.)

Note: When changing the lip shape, use a tapered lip brush and a concealer that simulates the natural coloring around the lipline. Recreate the lip shape by applying the concealer at the lipline. Every mouth has a natural light line surrounding the lip shape. Whenever you create a change in the shape of the mouth, this must be added to create a natural illusion. The light line adds dimension so that the lips look real and not placed on the face.

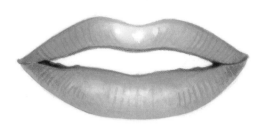

Flat Upper Lip

Using the edge of a lip brush, apply concealer to the upper lip; then create a curved shape with a brush above the natural lipline. Next powder the lips and add definition using a natural lipliner; fill with desired color.

Oversized Upper Lip

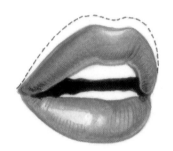

Apply concealer and powder the lips; then line the inside of the upper lip and the outside of the lower lip to create balance. Highlight the lower lip using a paler shade of matching lipcolor.

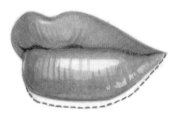

Oversized Bottom Lip

Reverse the technique described above.

Wrinkled Lips

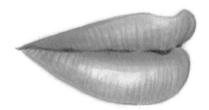

Use plenty of shine to reflect light out of the lines. Try to keep the product toward the inner part of the mouth to avoid color bleeding outside of lines.

Note: If a client has a deep nasolabial fold (laugh line), apply the lipliner to arch inward toward the mouth. If the liner is arched outward (toward the lines), it will bring attention to the area. In addition, for clients with a full cheek area, arching the liner inward will help to give the illusion of less weight.

the makeovers

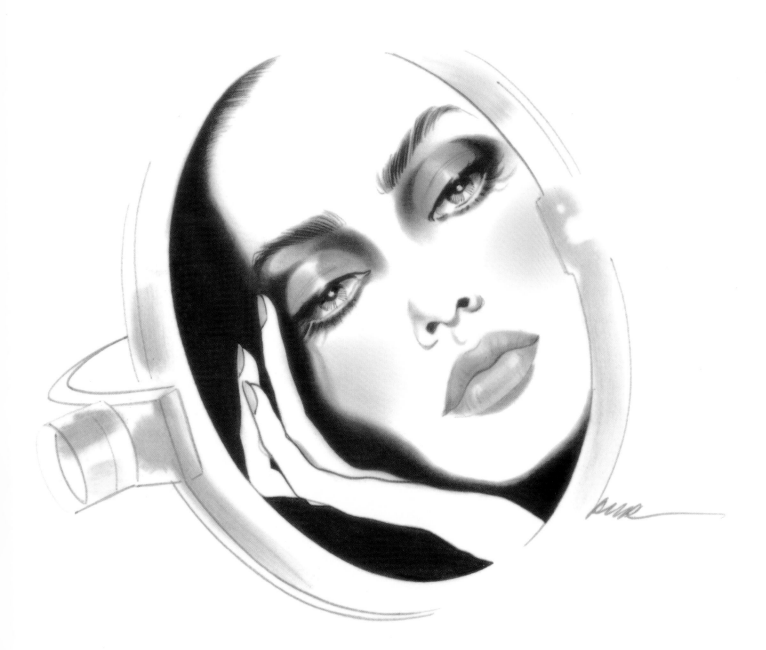

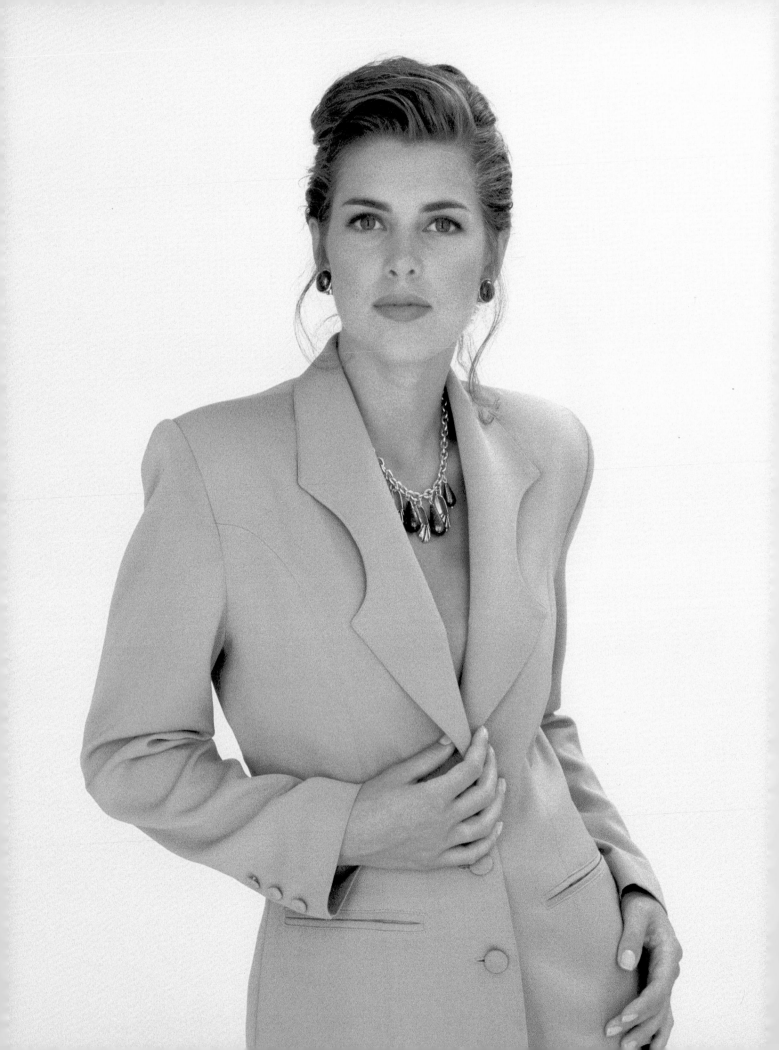

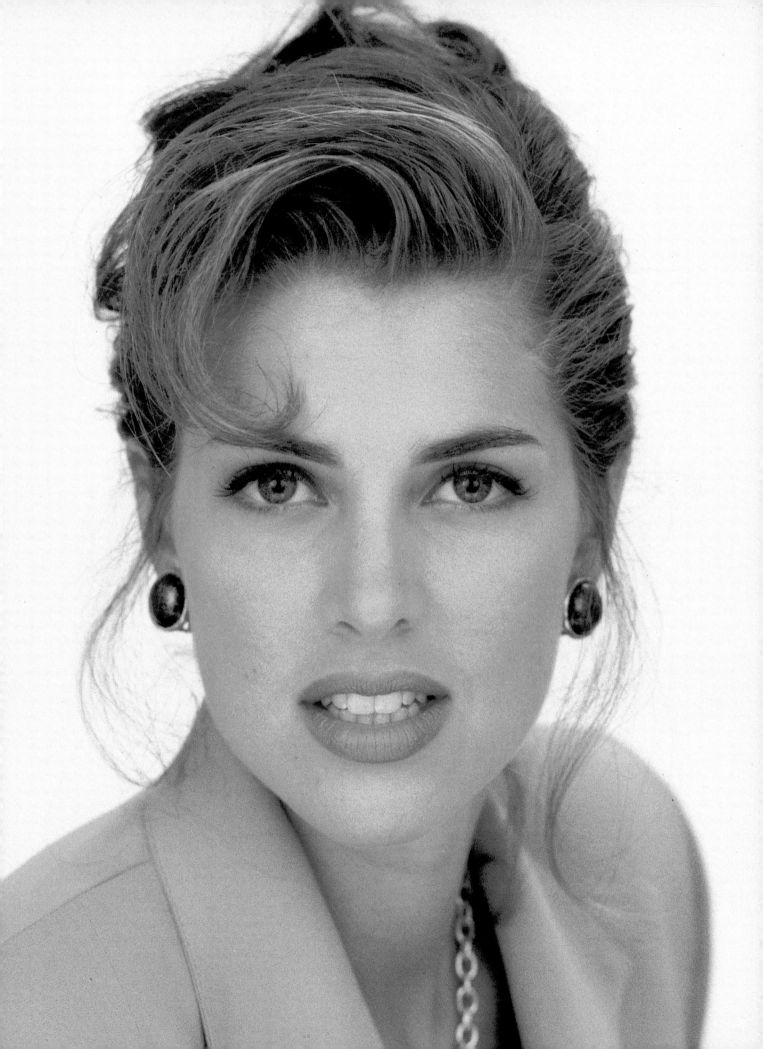

step-by-step techniques to a makeover

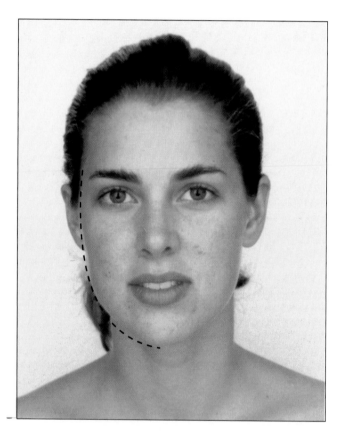

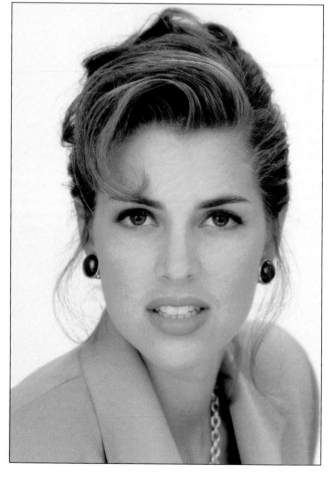

OBSERVATIONS

Face Shape: Oval

Skin Type: Normal to oily

Skintone: Sallow with blemishes on cheek area

Eye Color: Blue

Problem Areas: Discoloration beneath eyes; uneven skin tone; uneven eyebrows

Best Features: Blue eyes; full lips; nice facial structure

Model: Kristin
Hair: René/Peter's Place, Great Neck, New York
Makeup: Pamela Taylor, New York City
Accessories: The Accessory Shop, New York City
Photography: Christian Pollard, New York City
Still Photos: David Hamsley, New York City

Step 1: A yellow-based concealer is mixed and applied to under-eye discolorations and on blemishes in the cheek area and sides of the nostrils.

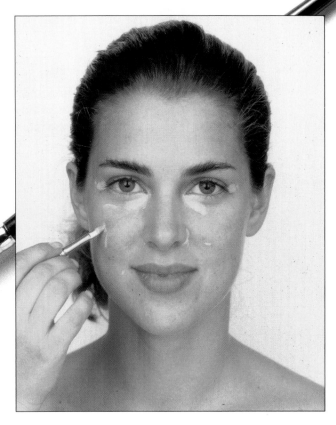

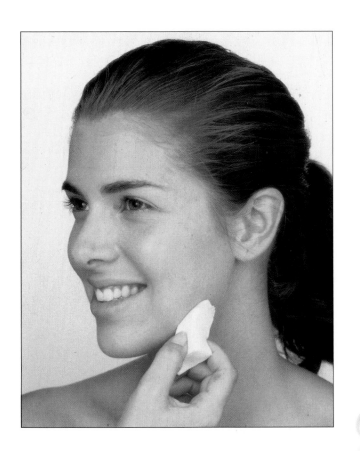

Step 2: Natural beige cream photography base is applied using a sponge wedge to even the skintone.

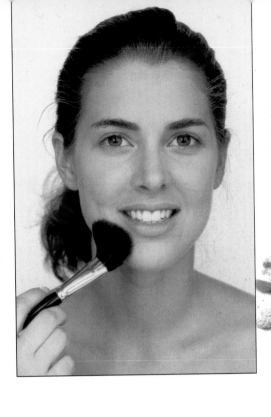

Step 3: A loose, neutral, transparent powder is applied to set the foundation.

Step 4: Soleil (reddish brown) and natural peach powder blusher are mixed and gently applied to the cheeks, forehead, and chin.

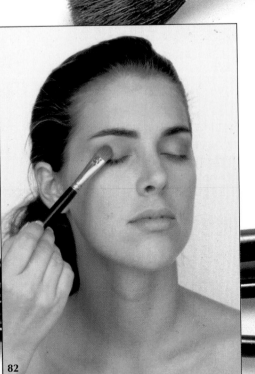

Step 5: Following the brow shaping, soft cerise and pearl shadows are blended onto the lid, and brown shadow gently contours the eye.

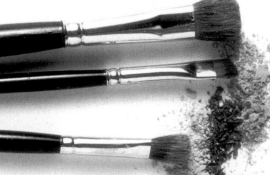

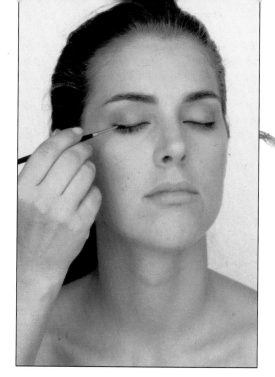

Step 6: Using a fine liner brush, soft black cake eyeliner defines the upper lashline.

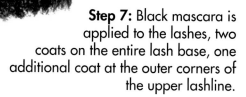

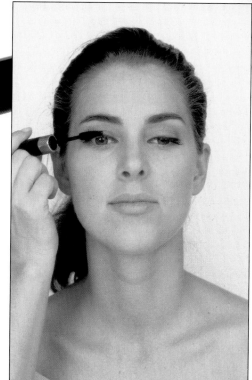

Step 7: Black mascara is applied to the lashes, two coats on the entire lash base, one additional coat at the outer corners of the upper lashline.

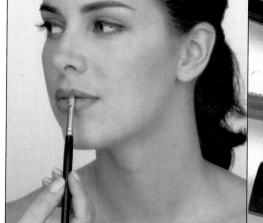

Step 8: Lips are lined with a natural brown-toned pencil, then filled with a complimenting lipstick shade.

After completing the application, all makeup is blended to finish the look.

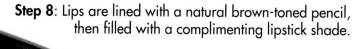

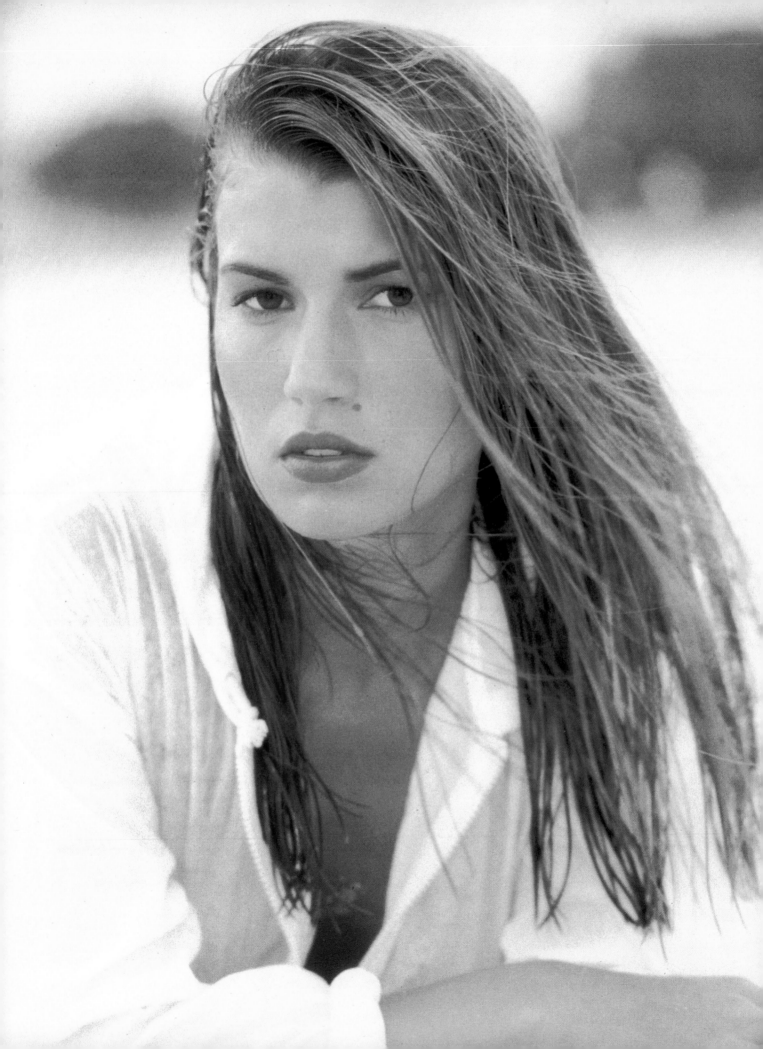

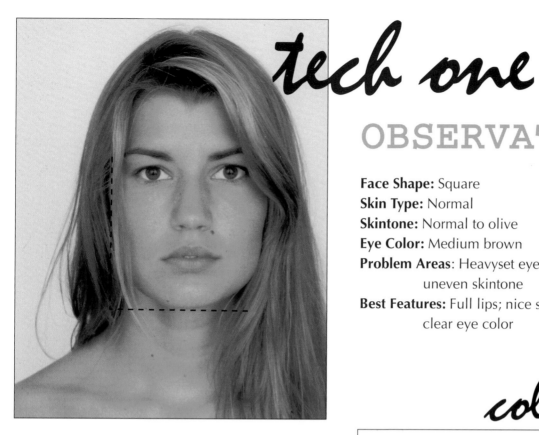

tech one

OBSERVATIONS

Face Shape: Square
Skin Type: Normal
Skintone: Normal to olive
Eye Color: Medium brown
Problem Areas: Heavyset eyelid;
uneven skintone
Best Features: Full lips; nice skin texture;
clear eye color

color key

Model: Aimi
Agency: Irene Marie, Florida
Hair: Shai/Yellow Strawberry Salon, Florida
Makeup: Pamela Taylor, New York City
Photography: Christian Pollard, New York City

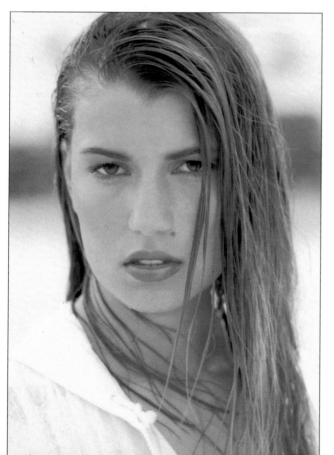

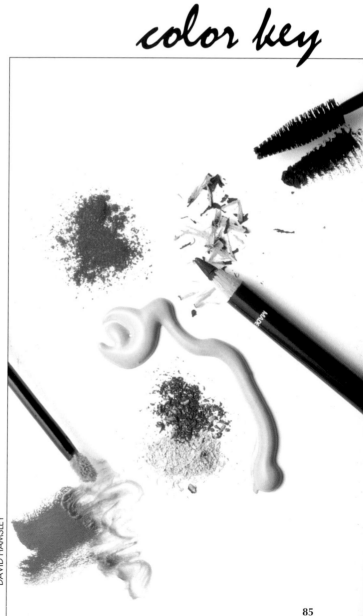

DAVID HAMSLEY

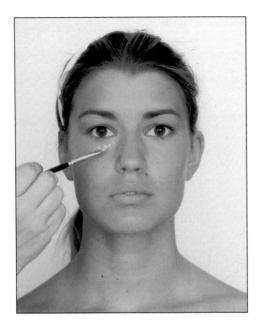

Step 1: Yellow/beige cream concealer is blended on the sides of nose and beneath the eyes to diminish the discolored areas.

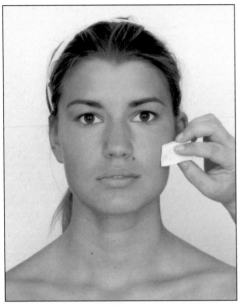

Step 2: Natural tan and beige liquid foundations are blended and applied using a moistened wedge to even the skintone.

Step 3: Loose, waterproof, transparent powder is pressed onto the base to set the makeup and remove excess shine.

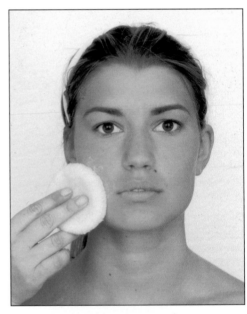

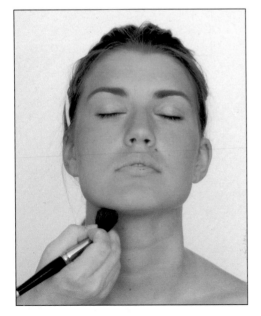

Step 4: The jawline is given the illusion of balance by applying a shading powder onto the lower right jaw.

Step 5: Soft matte red blush is gently swept onto the cheekbone and around the chin, nose, and temple areas.

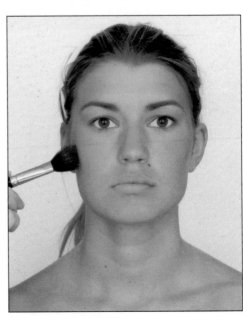

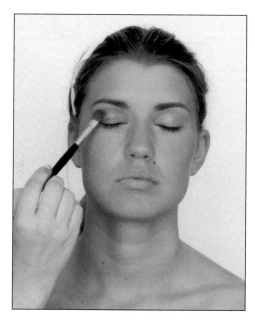

Step 6: Golden brown shadow is applied over the lid using a chiseled fluff brush; matte cream is used to highlight the brow bone.

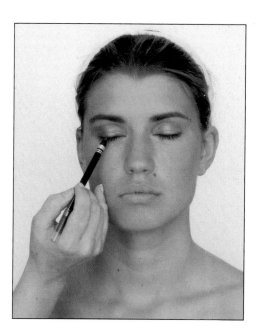

Step 7: Deep rich brown waterproof pencil liner is applied to the upper lashline to add definition to the lash base.

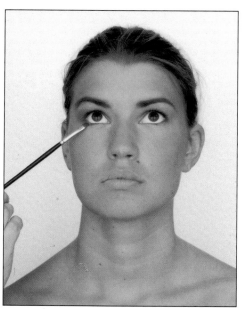

Step 8: A rich brown pencil liner is softly applied to the outer corner of the eyes with an angle brush.

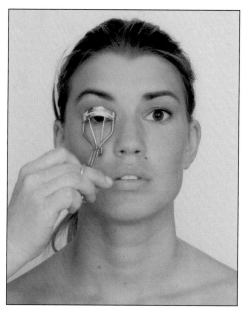

Step 9: Lashes are curled; then black/brown mascara is applied.

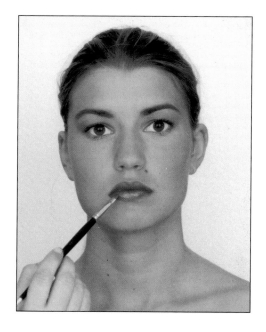

Step 10: Using an angle-tip brush, sheer sienna lipcolor is applied, then blotted to reduce shine.

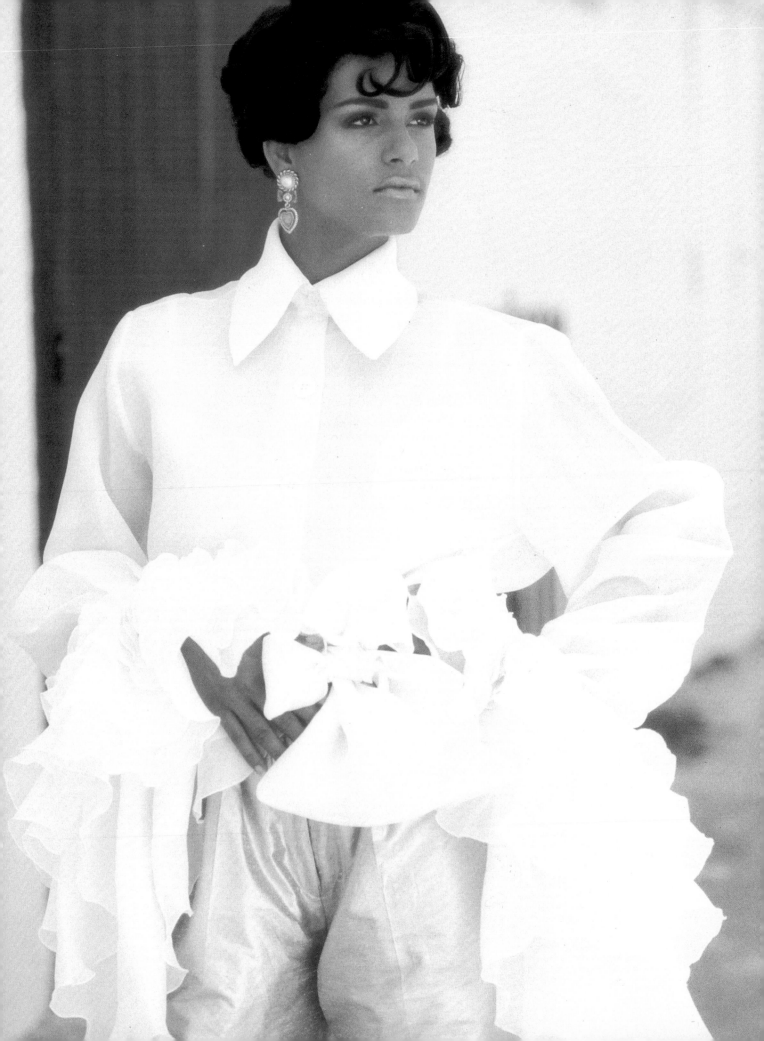

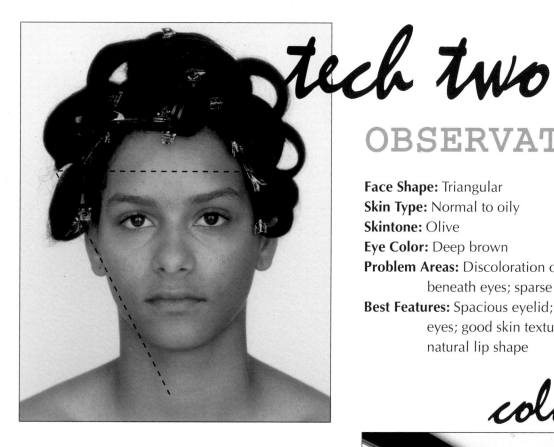

tech two

OBSERVATIONS

Face Shape: Triangular
Skin Type: Normal to oily
Skintone: Olive
Eye Color: Deep brown
Problem Areas: Discoloration on skin; recession beneath eyes; sparse eyebrows
Best Features: Spacious eyelid; almond-shaped eyes; good skin texture; well-defined, natural lip shape

color key

Model: Key
Agency: Powers, Florida
Hair: Shai/Yellow Strawberry Salon, Florida
Makeup: Pamela Taylor, New York City
Photography: Christian Pollard, New York City

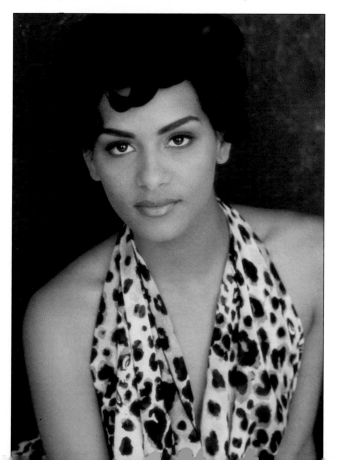

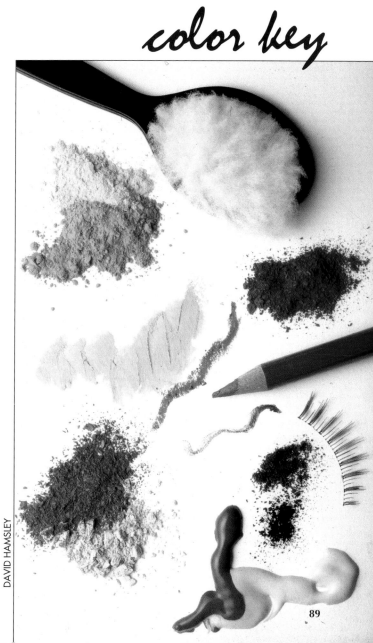

DAVID HAMSLEY

89

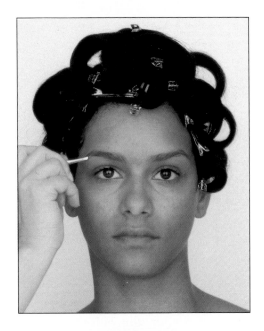

Step 1: To shape the brows, excess hair is removed from the center of the eyebrows and under the brow.

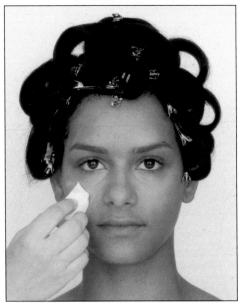

Step 2: Following concealer, cream foundation is custom blended and applied with a wedge to even out the skintone.

Step 3: Ochre and beige translucent powders are blended and buffed onto the skin to remove excess shine and to set the base.

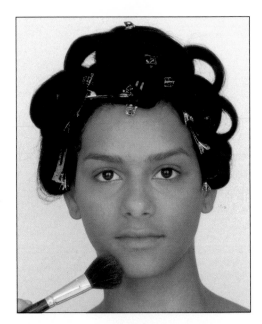

Step 4: Brows are filled and arched using a deep brown and black blended shadow on a moistened angular shadow brush.

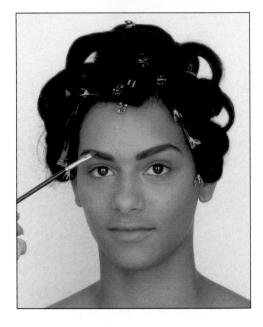

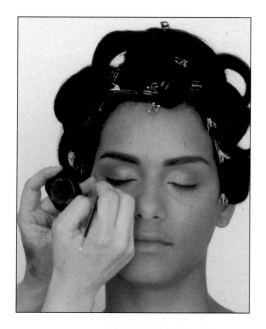

Step 5: Pearl cream highlight and reddish brown contour shadow are used to shade and define the eyes, followed by black cake eyeliner applied to the upper lash base.

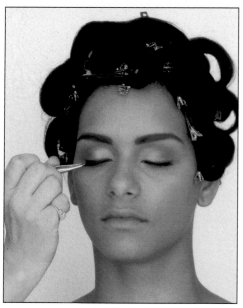

Step 6: Strip lashes are measured to fit and applied to the base of the upper lashline.

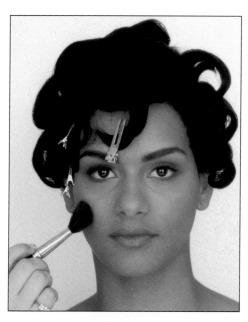

Step 7: Soft russett blush is applied to accentuate the cheekbones.

Step 8: Mocha lip pencil is used to define the lips, followed by sheer golden lipstick to fill in. (**Note**: Pure gold lip color is added for an on-location photo.)

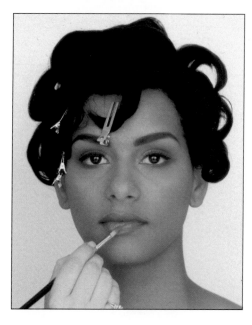

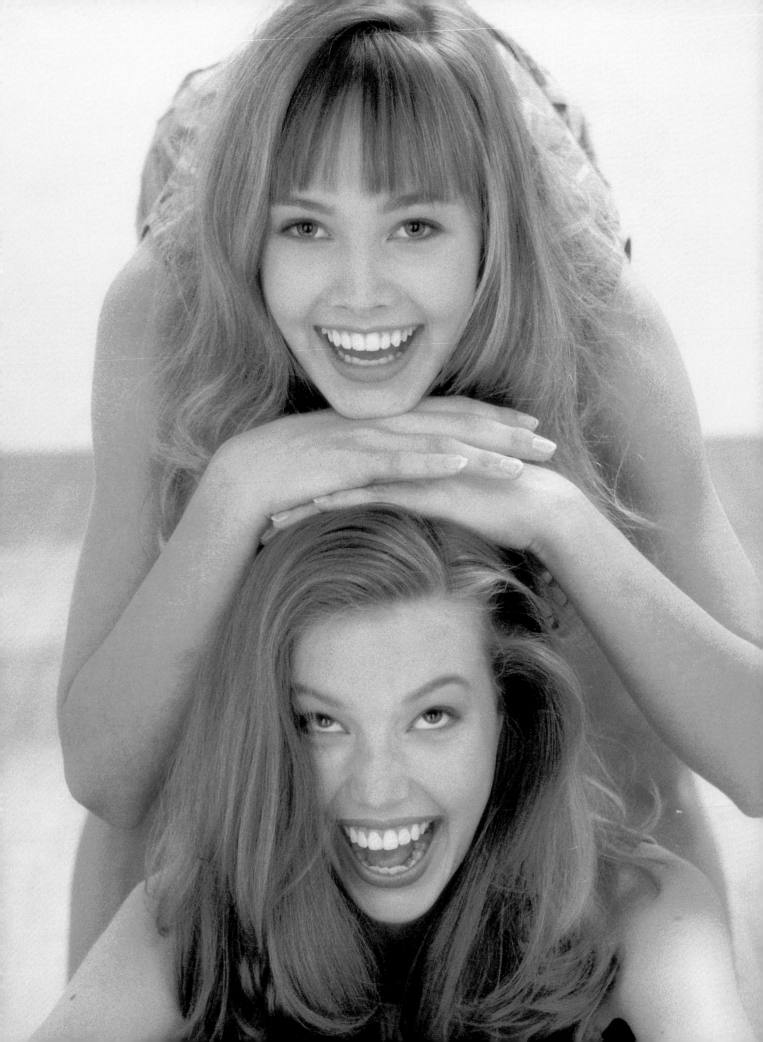

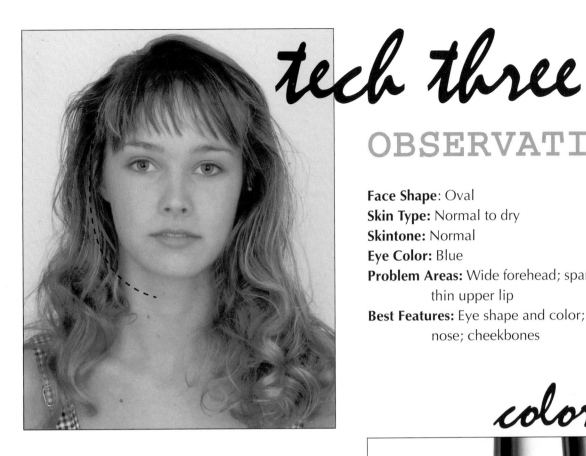

tech three

OBSERVATIONS

Face Shape: Oval
Skin Type: Normal to dry
Skintone: Normal
Eye Color: Blue
Problem Areas: Wide forehead; sparse brows;
       thin upper lip
Best Features: Eye shape and color;
       nose; cheekbones

color key

Model: Ashley
Agency: Boldt, New York City
Hair: René/Peter's Place, Great Neck, New York
Makeup: Pamela Taylor, New York City
Photography: Christian Pollard, New York City

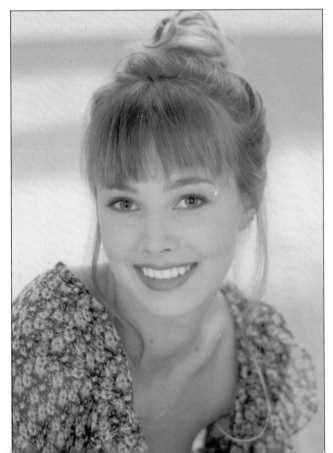

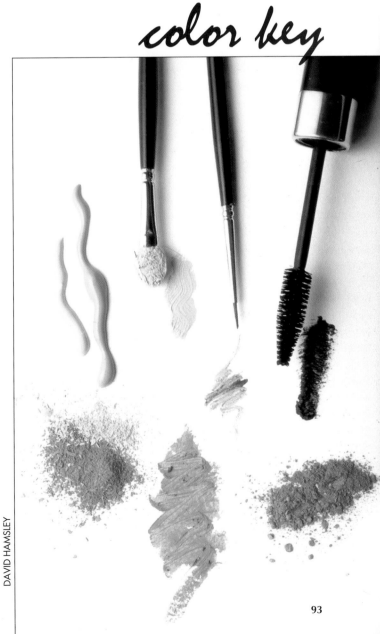

DAVID HAMSLEY

93

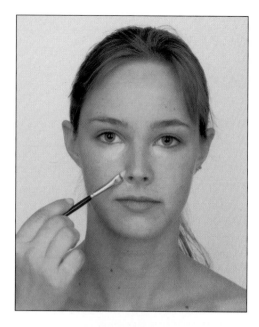

Step 1: Applied to a flat sable brush, yellow-based concealer is used to cover redness around the nostrils and under the eyes.

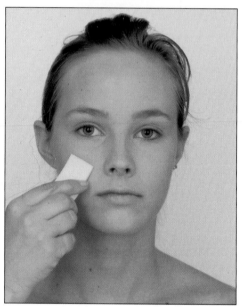

Step 2: Light and medium beige water-based foundations are blended and applied to even the skintone.

Step 3: Loose transparent powder is buffed to remove shine from the face and to set the foundation.

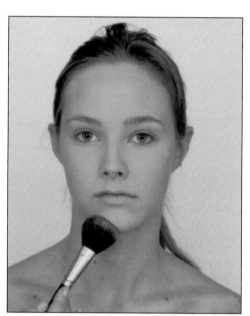

Step 4: Matte peach blush is softened with beige powder and applied to accentuate the cheekbones.

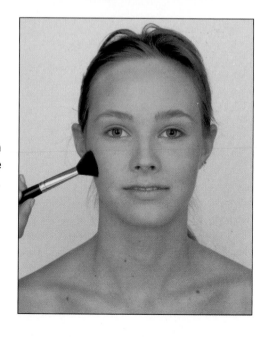

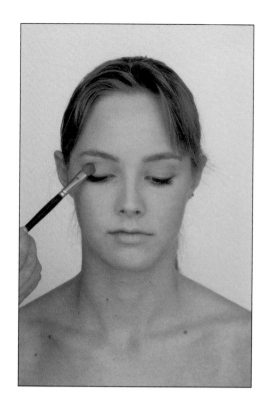

Step 5: Following an application of black/brown cake eyeliner, matte ginger shadow tints the eyelids.

Step 6: Lashes are coated with black mascara and brushed to create a natural look.

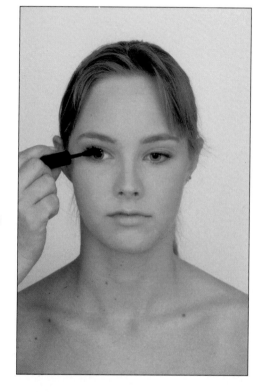

Step 7: Lips are moistened with balm and filled with a matte medium peach lipcolor.

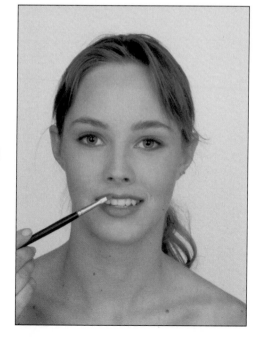

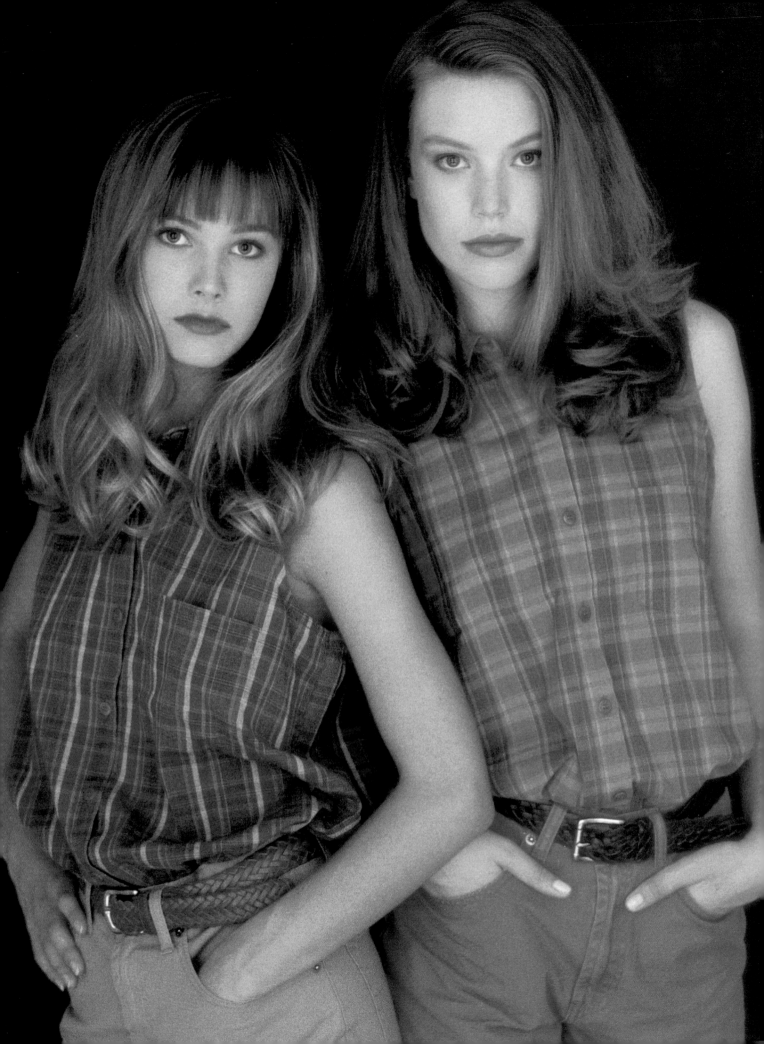

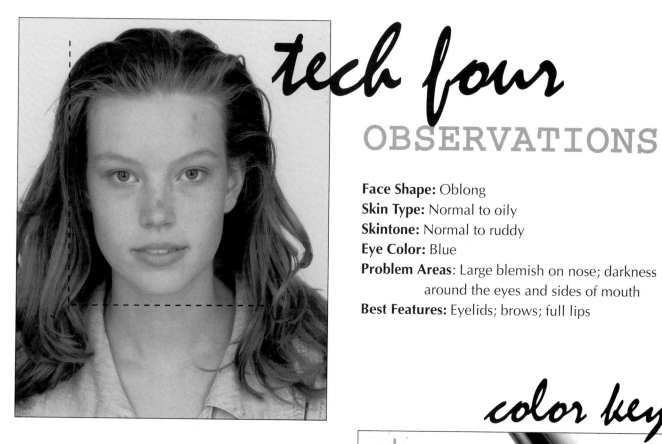

tech four

OBSERVATIONS

Face Shape: Oblong
Skin Type: Normal to oily
Skintone: Normal to ruddy
Eye Color: Blue
Problem Areas: Large blemish on nose; darkness
 around the eyes and sides of mouth
Best Features: Eyelids; brows; full lips

Model: Jessica
Agency: Boldt, New York City
Hair: René/ Peter's Place, Great Neck, New York
Makeup: Pamela Taylor, New York City
Photography: Christian Pollard, New York City

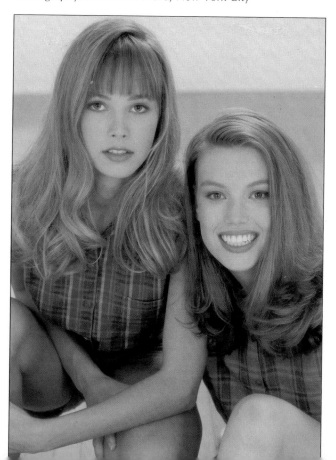

color key

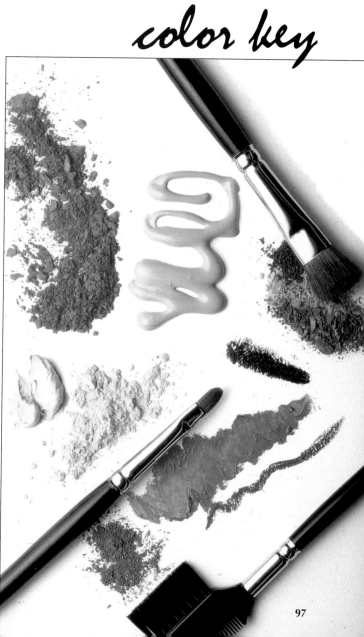

DAVID HAMSLEY

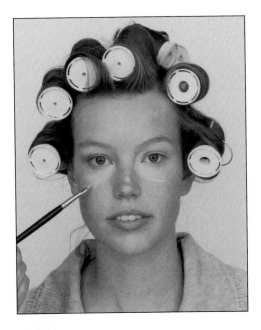

Step 1: Corrective concealer is applied to the dark undereye discoloration and directly onto the blemish at the bridge of the nose.

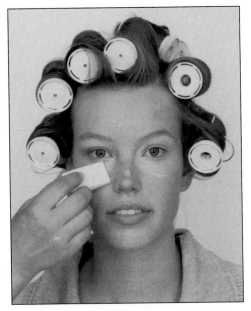

Step 2: Cream make-up that has been applied to a moistened wedge is used to even the skintone.

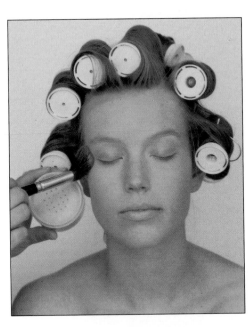

Step 3: Translucent powder is applied to the entire face and buffed with a sable powder brush.

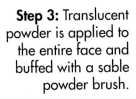

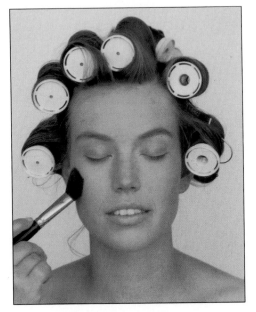

Step 4: Mauve cheek color adds soft definition.

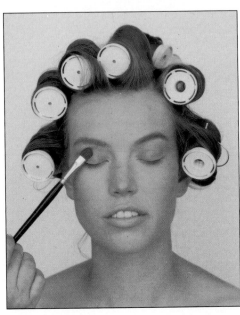

Step 5: Amethyst demi-pearl shadow is applied to the upper eyelid followed by a cream-colored highlight at the brow bone.

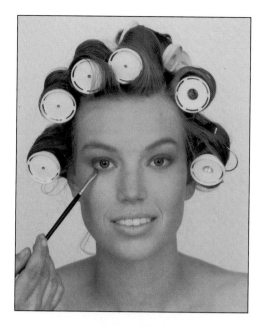

Step 6: Grey shadow is applied to the outer half of the lower lash base and blended using an angular brush.

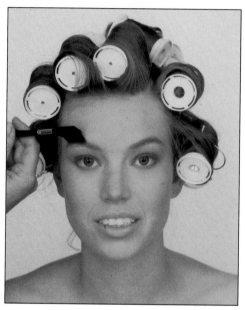

Step 7: Eyebrows are softly defined using a light ash brown powdered shadow.

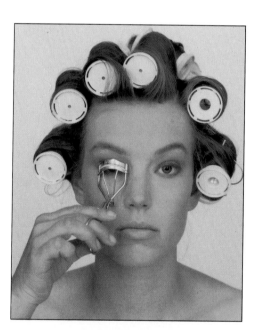

Step 8: Lashes are curled at the base to lift the eyes.

Step 9: After soft plum lipliner has been applied to define the lips, sheer plum lipcolor is added.

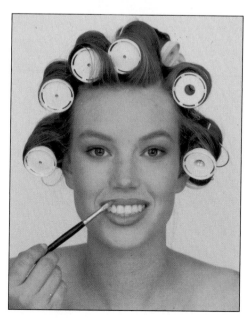

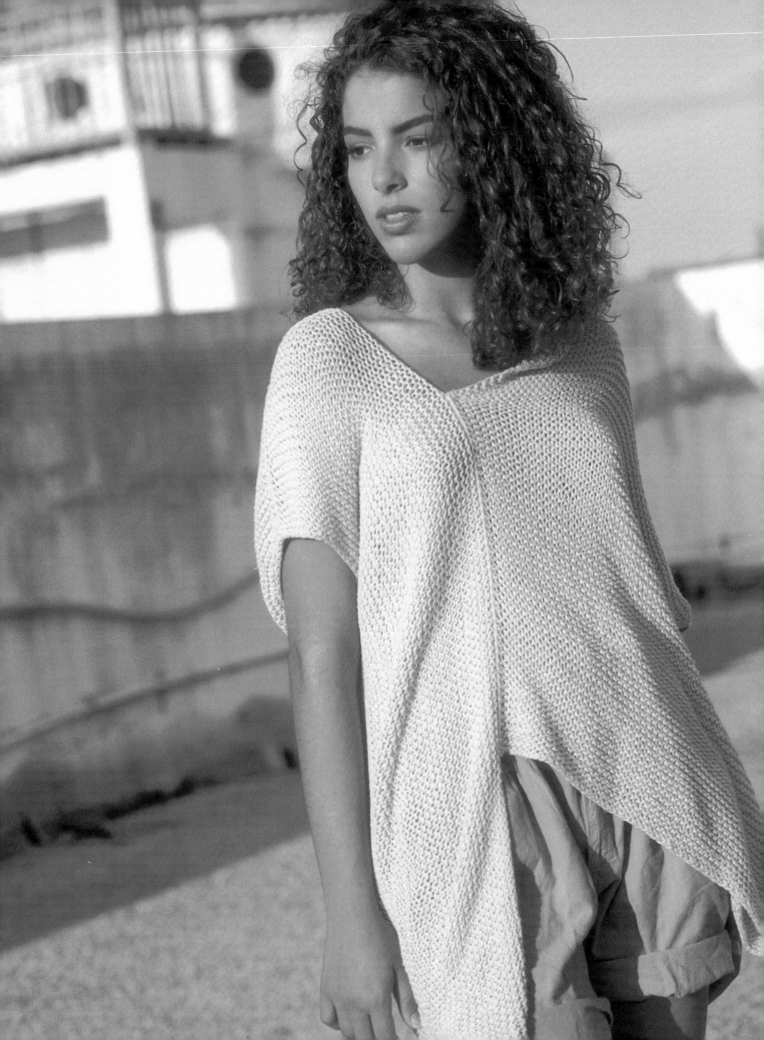

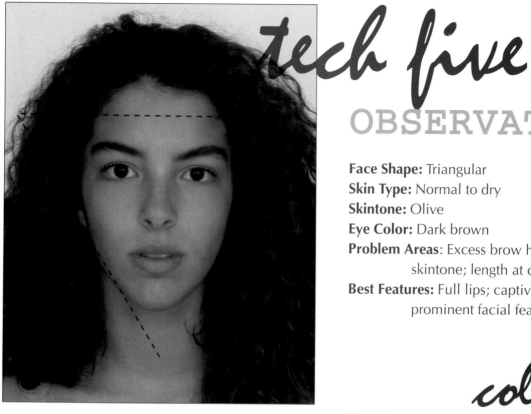

tech five
OBSERVATIONS

Face Shape: Triangular
Skin Type: Normal to dry
Skintone: Olive
Eye Color: Dark brown
Problem Areas: Excess brow hair; uneven skintone; length at chin
Best Features: Full lips; captivating eyes; prominent facial features

color key

Model: Nanette
Agency: Powers, Florida
Hair: Shai/Yellow Strawberry Salon, Florida
Makeup: Pamela Taylor, New York City
Photography: Christian Pollard, New York City

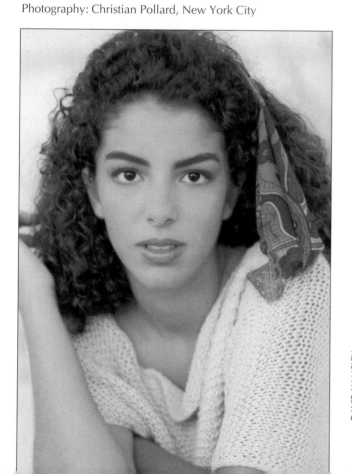

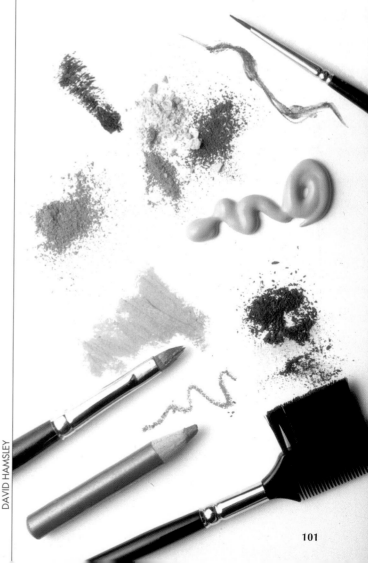

DAVID HAMSLEY

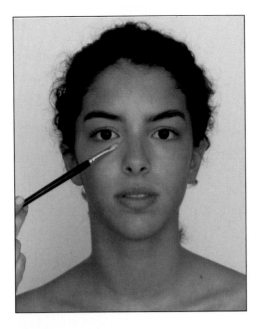

Step 1: Concealer is applied to correct undereye discoloration, then blended using a flat sable brush.

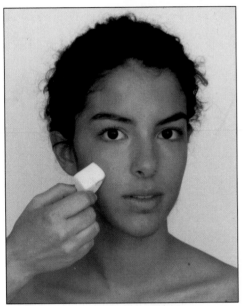

Step 2: Water-based foundation is blended to match the skintone and is applied to the face using a latex wedge.

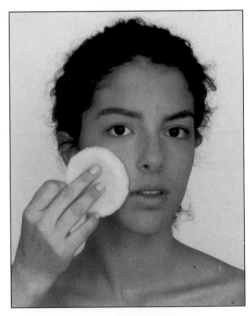

Step 3: Transparent rice powder is applied to a powder puff and pressed onto the foundation to set the makeup.

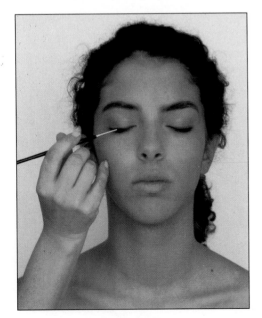

Step 4: Following an application of matte ginger and demi-pearl light brown shadow, dark brown cake liner is applied to the lashline and beneath the eye to create definition.

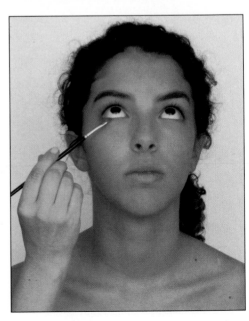

Step 5: Liner is softened using a tapered angular brush to achieve a blended effect in the upper and lower lashlines.

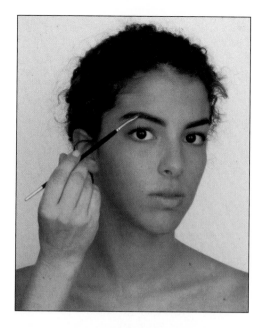

Step 6: After applying soft black mascara to the lashes, rich brown shadow is applied to an angular brow brush and is used to fill and define the brows.

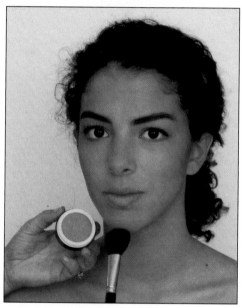

Step 7: To create the illusion of a less prominent chin, contour powder is applied to the tip and blended.

Step 8: Soft peach blush is applied to the apple of the cheeks, achieving a natural glow.

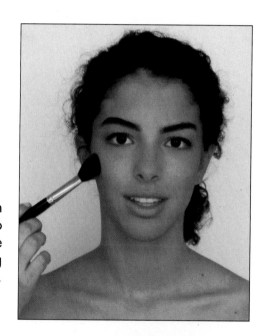

Step 9: Natural lipliner adds definition to the lip shape and is filled with sheer brown spice lip color.

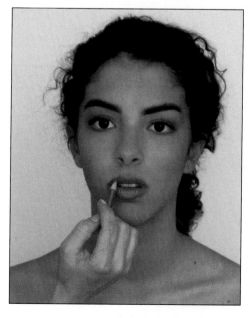

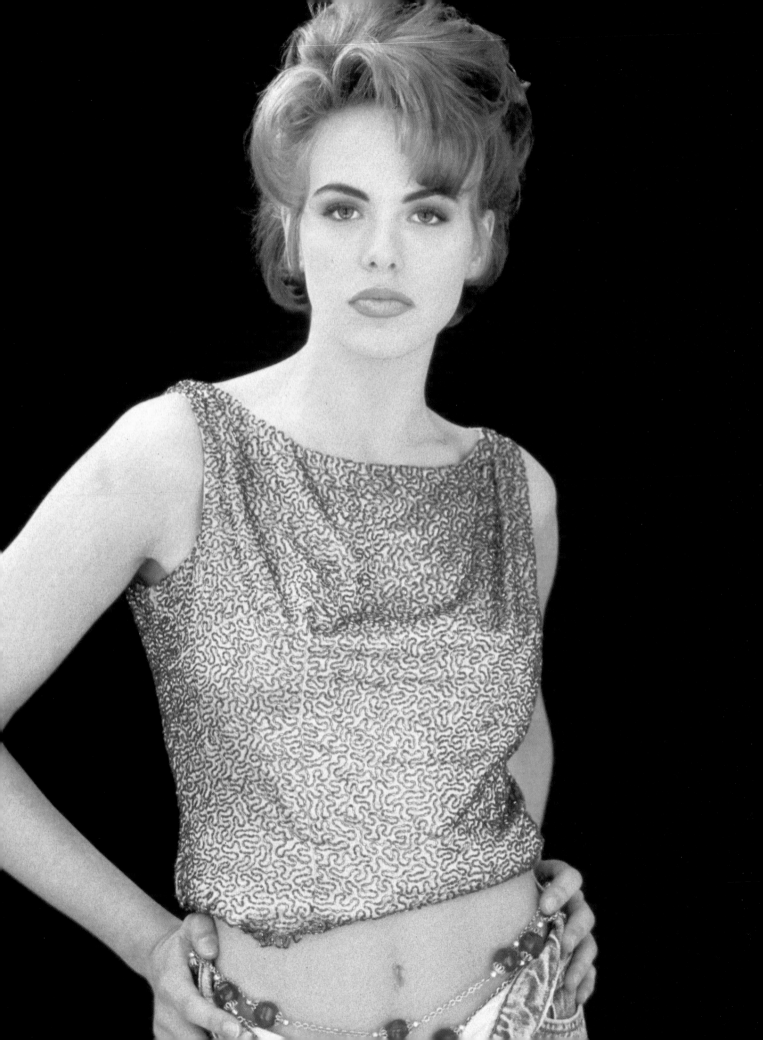

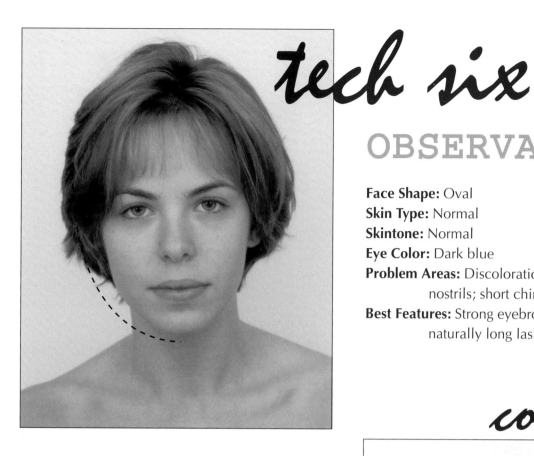

tech six

OBSERVATIONS

Face Shape: Oval
Skin Type: Normal
Skintone: Normal
Eye Color: Dark blue
Problem Areas: Discoloration around
nostrils; short chin
Best Features: Strong eyebrows; full lips;
naturally long lashes

color key

Model: Suzanne
Agency: 6.7.8, New York City
Hair: Eve/Peter's Place, Great Neck, New York
Makeup: Pamela Taylor, New York City
Photography: Christian Pollard, New York City

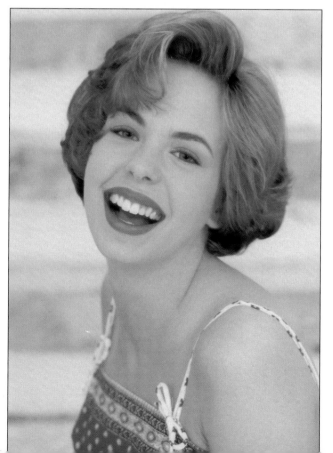

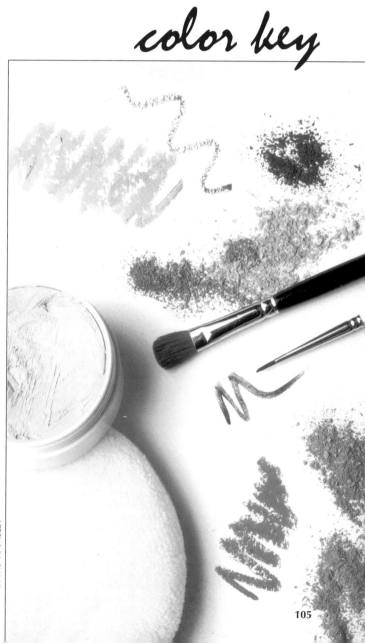

DAVID HAMSLEY

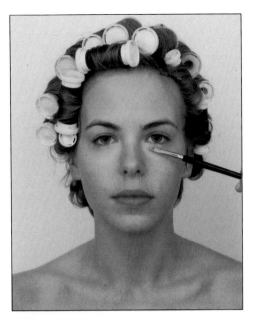

Step 1: Concealer is applied wih a flat brush to recessed area under the eyes.

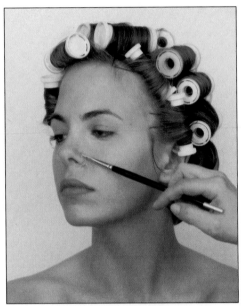

Step 2: Using a pointed sable brush, yellow cream toner removes discoloration on the sides of nose.

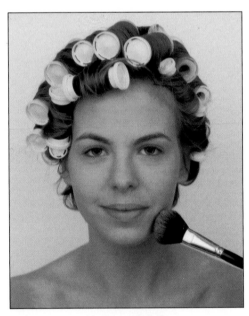

Step 3: Following the application of a sheer beige water-based foundation, translucent powder is dusted over the face to set the cream makeup.

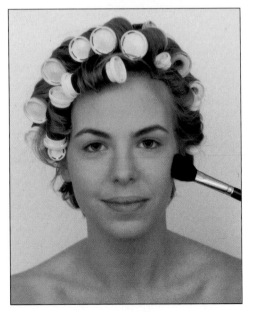

Step 4: Warm matte peach cheek color enhances the face.

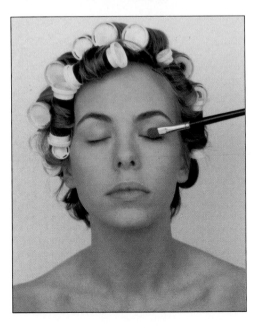

Step 5: A mixture of peach and ginger shadow shades the lower eyelid followed by matte cream shadow to highlight the area beneath the browbone.

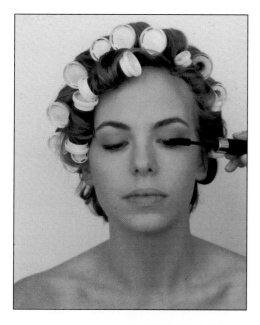

Step 6: Black mascara coats the natural lashes to define the eye.

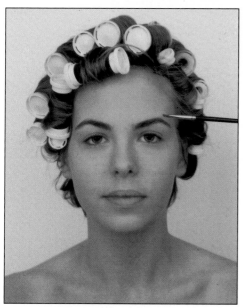

Step 7: Sable powder fills the brow for definition.

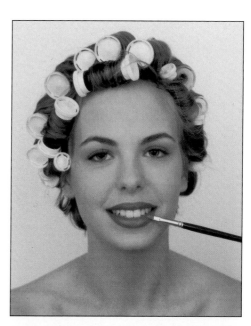

Step 8: Matte pink-coral lipstick shades the natural lipline and is blotted to reduce excess shine.

Step 9: A change of lipcolor to a soft golden brown creates another look.

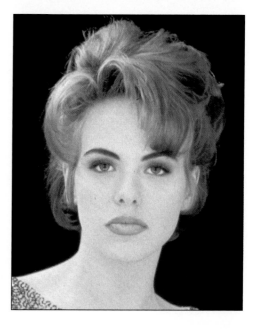

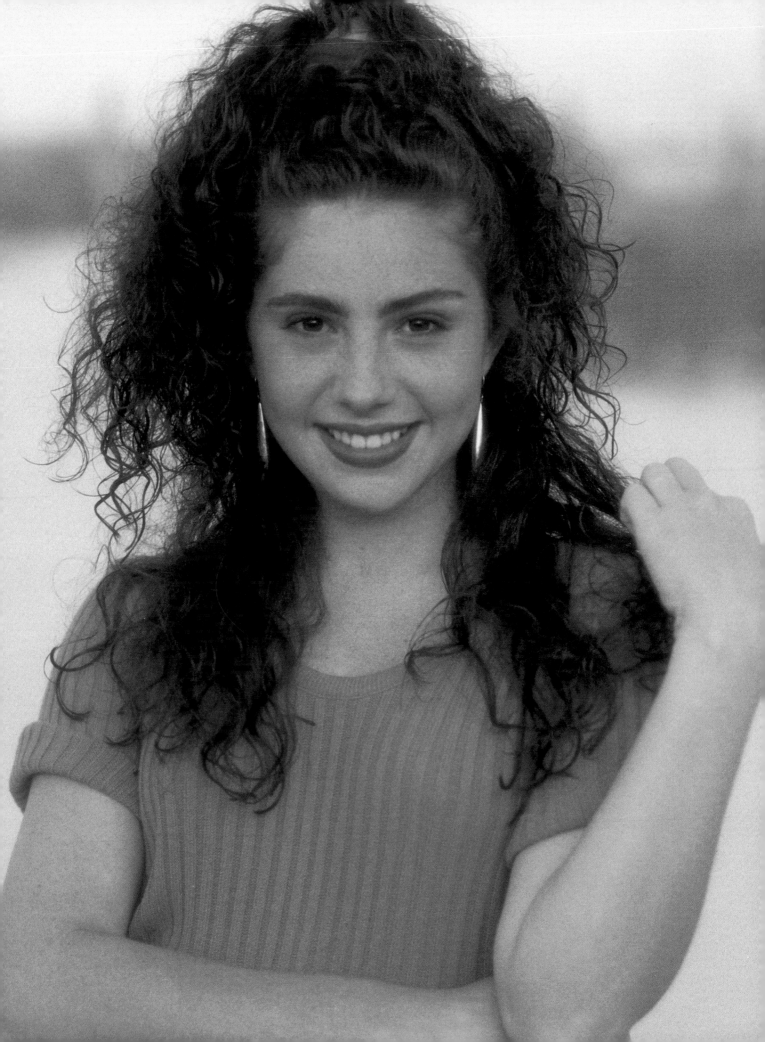

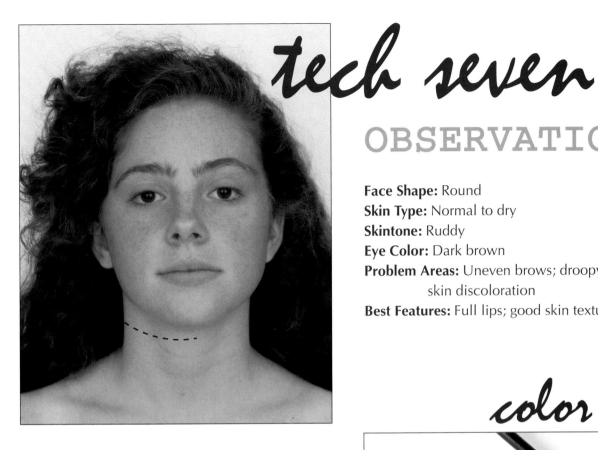

tech seven

OBSERVATIONS

Face Shape: Round
Skin Type: Normal to dry
Skintone: Ruddy
Eye Color: Dark brown
Problem Areas: Uneven brows; droopy eyelids; skin discoloration
Best Features: Full lips; good skin texture

color key

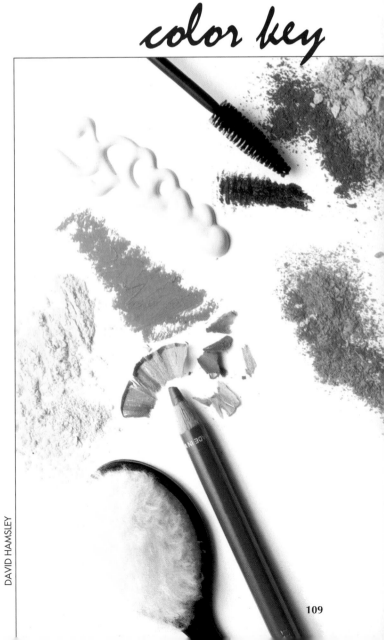

Model: Aimara
Agency: Powers, Florida
Hair: Shai/Yellow Strawberry Salon, Florida
Makeup: Pamela Taylor, New York City
Photography: Christian Pollard, New York City

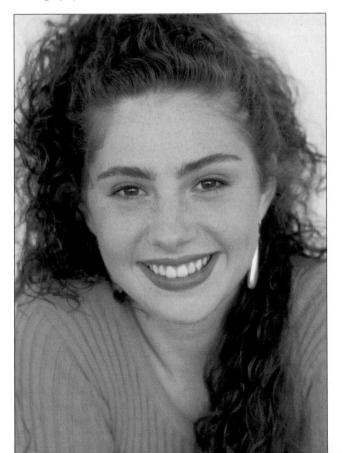

DAVID HAMSLEY

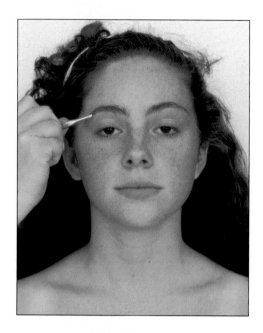

Step 1: Eyebrows are tweezed in the direction of the natural hair growth, removing unwanted hair at the center of the eyes and beneath the brows.

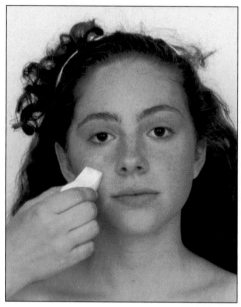

Step 2: After highlighting recessed areas under the eyes, a sheer water-based foundation balances the skintone.

Step 3: Translucent powder applied to a velour powder puff is pressed over the foundation and buffed to set the makeup.

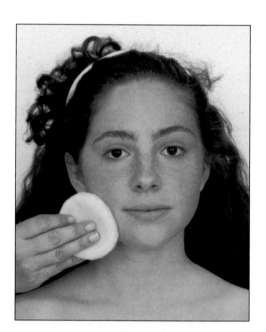

Step 4: Pale yellow shadow is swept over the inner corner of the lids; then natural clay shadow is wrapped around the contour of the eye and softly applied at the lower lashline.

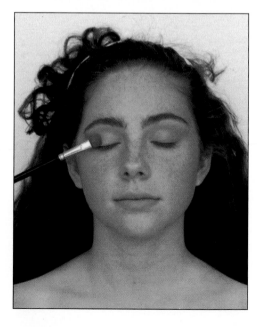

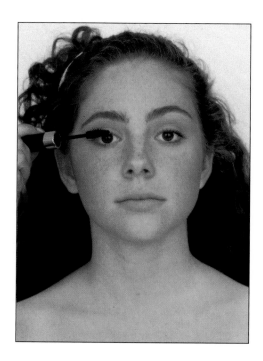

Step 5: After the lashes have been curled, they are coated with black/brown mascara and combed for a natural look.

Step 6: Matte coral-peach blush gently adds color to the cheeks, forehead, and chin.

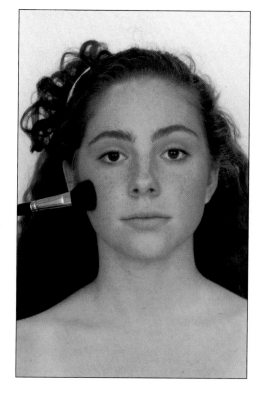

Step 7: Lips are defined using a ginger lip pencil and filled in with a coral cream lipcolor.

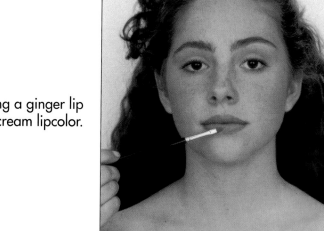

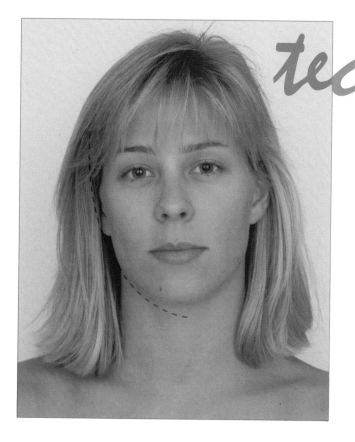

tech eight

OBSERVATIONS

Face Shape: Oval
Skin Type: Normal
Skintone: Normal
Eye Color: Deep blue
Problem Areas: Fullness at jaw and cheeks; discoloration beneath eyes
Best Features: Forehead; eyebrows; and lips

Model: Lynlee
Agency: Act 1, Miami, Florida
Hair: Shai/Yellow Strawberry Salon, Florida
Makeup: Pamela Taylor, New York City
Photography: Christian Pollard, New York City

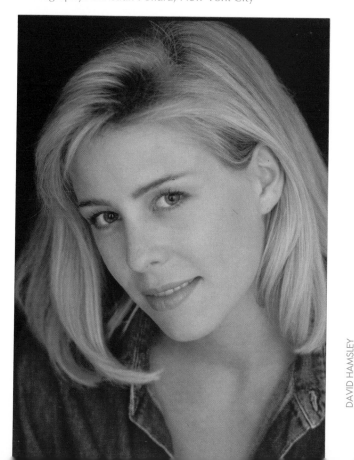

color key

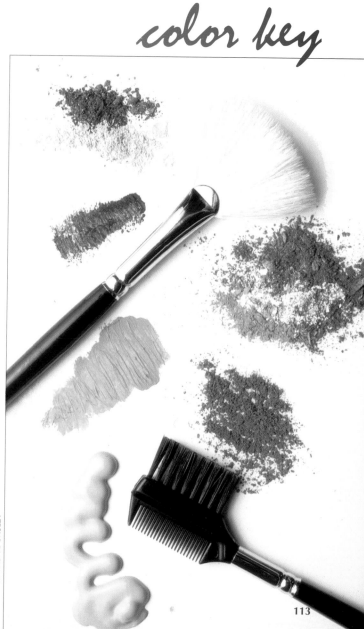

DAVID HAMSLEY

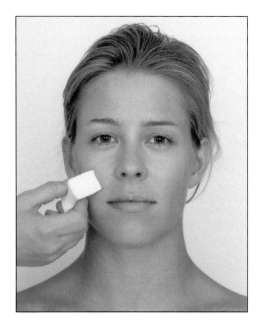

Step 1: Cream concealer is applied to lift out recessed discoloration under the eyes; then a medium beige cream foundation is blended to even the skintone.

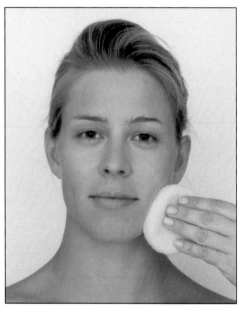

Step 2: Loose transparent powder applied to a velour powder puff is pressed onto the base, which sets the makeup.

Step 3: Pure white matte powder is applied to highlight the cheekbone.

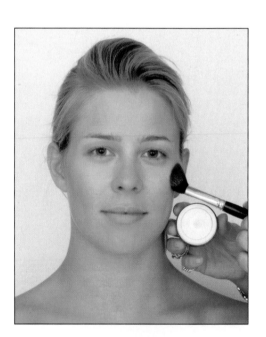

Step 4: Natural peach and tan powders are blended and applied to the cheek, nose, and forehead to give the illusion of a healthy glow.

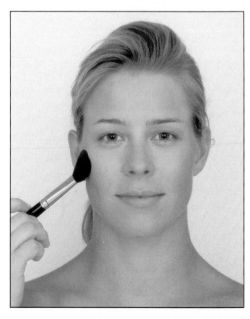

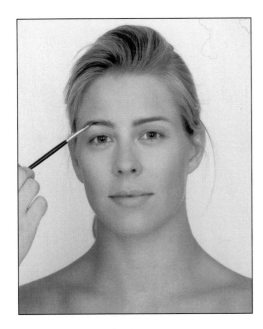

Step 5: Soft mocha powder fills and shapes the brows.

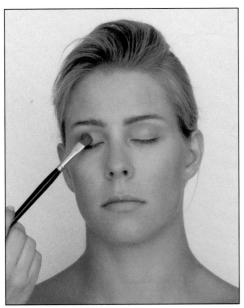

Step 6: A fluff brush is used to apply soft plum demi-pearl shadow over the entire lid; natural cream matte powder is used to highlight the browbone.

Step 7: Black/brown mascara coats the lashes; the eyelid is gently lifted so that mascara can be closely applied to the lash base.

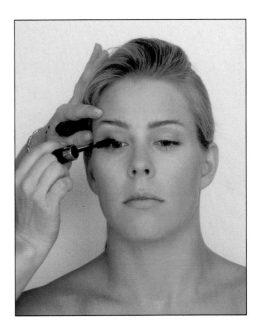

Step 8: Lips are moistened with a balm, followed by an application of mocha cream lipcolor.

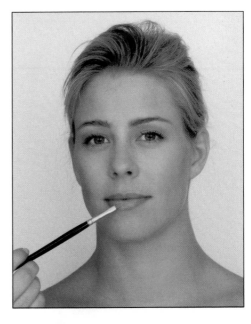

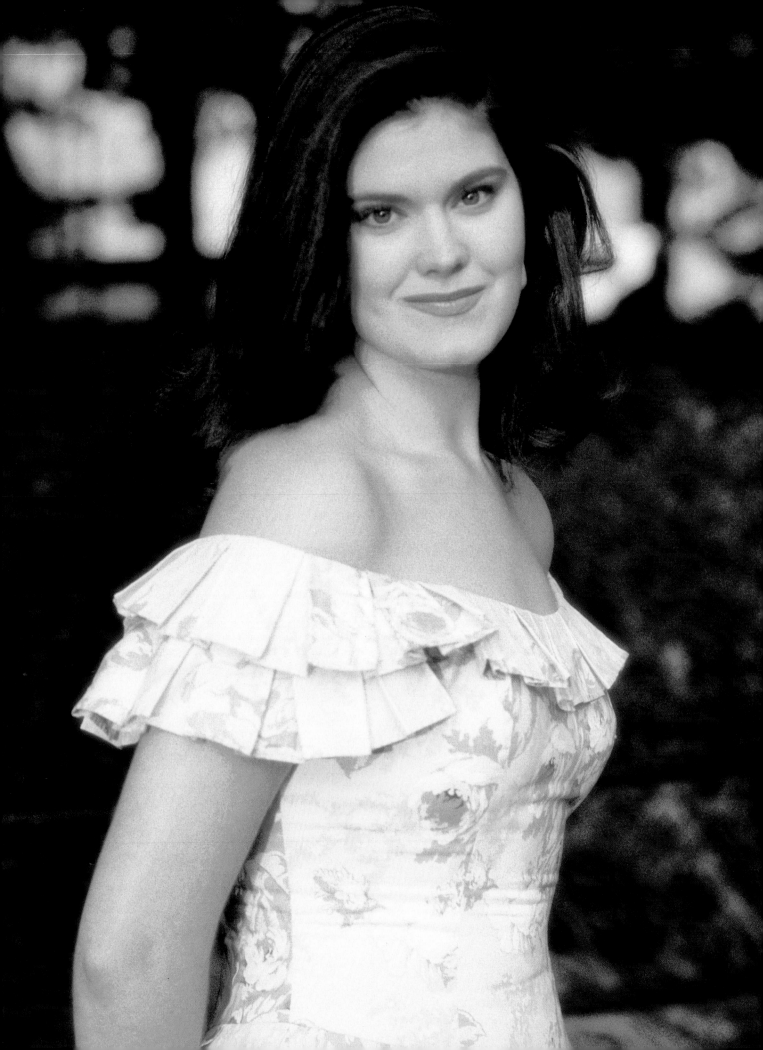

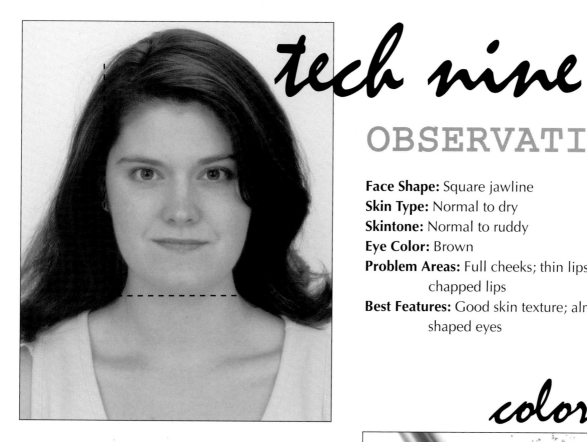

tech nine

OBSERVATIONS

Face Shape: Square jawline
Skin Type: Normal to dry
Skintone: Normal to ruddy
Eye Color: Brown
Problem Areas: Full cheeks; thin lips; chapped lips
Best Features: Good skin texture; almond-shaped eyes

Model: Andrea
Agency: Plus, New York City
Makeup: Pamela Taylor, New York City
Photography: Christian Pollard, New York City

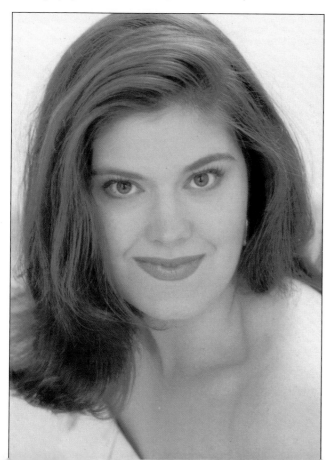

color key

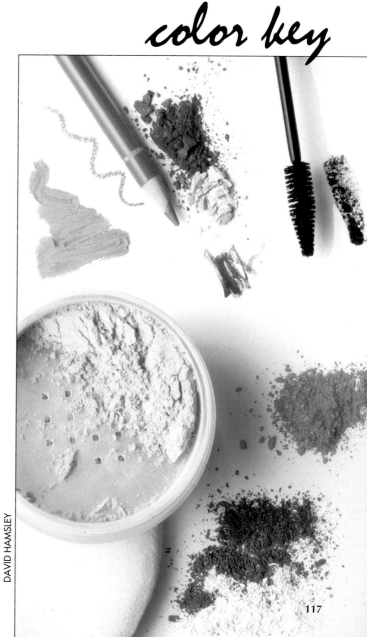

DAVID HAMSLEY

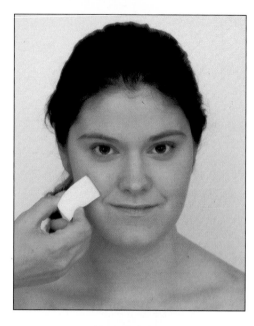

Step 1: A damp wedge is used to apply moisture-enriched foundation, to even the skintone.

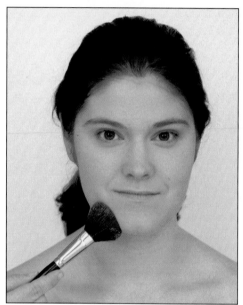

Step 2: Translucent powder a shade deeper than the foundation sets and deepens the skintone.

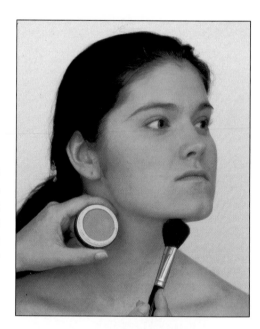

Step 3: An ash brown shading powder is applied to the area under the cheekbone and jawline, creating the illusion of a slimmer facial structure.

Step 4: Opposite the shading powder, matte white powder is applied to balance the face, followed by a sheer pink color on the cheekbone.

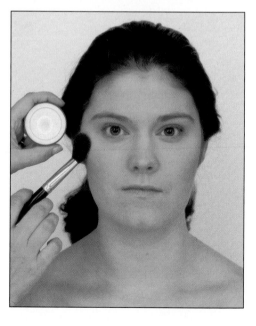

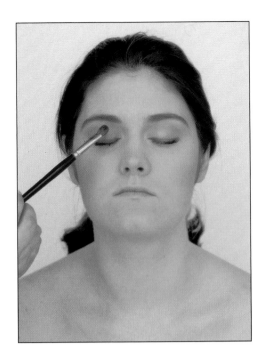

Step 5: Sable brown powder shadow is applied to upper lashline, and soft berry demi-pearl shadow is blended over the lid; brown shadow is then used on the outer half of the lower lashline and blended.

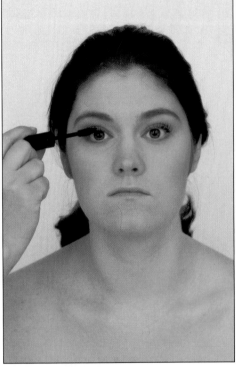

Step 6: Following brow shaping, lashes are curled and black mascara is applied to upper and lower lashes.

Step 7: Lips are overextended using a matte pink liner, then filled with a complimenting cream lip shade.

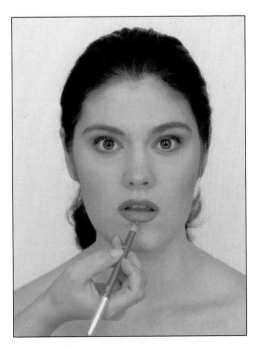

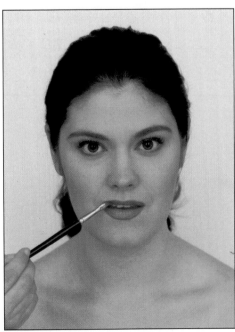

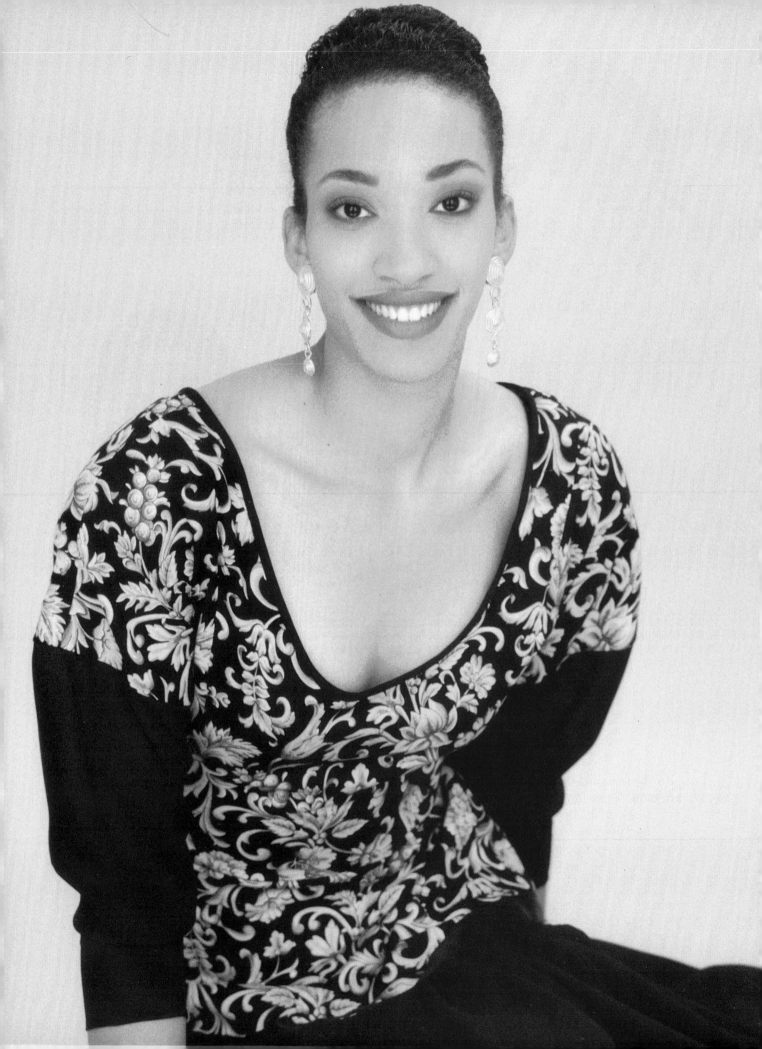

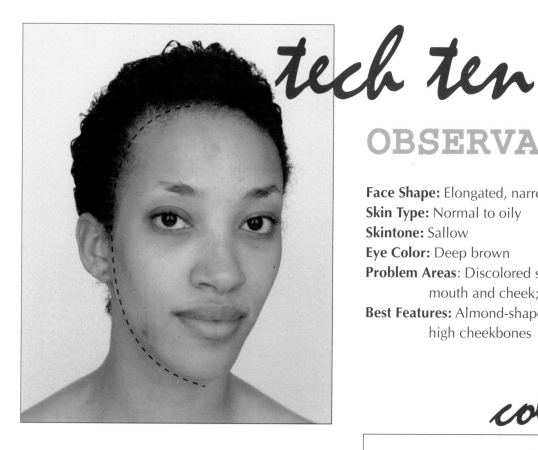

tech ten

OBSERVATIONS

Face Shape: Elongated, narrow
Skin Type: Normal to oily
Skintone: Sallow
Eye Color: Deep brown
Problem Areas: Discolored skin around
mouth and cheek; very sparse eyebrows
Best Features: Almond-shaped eyes;
high cheekbones

color key

Model: Deborah
Makeup: Pamela Taylor, New York City
Accessories: The Accessory Shop, New York City
Photography: Christian Pollard, New York City

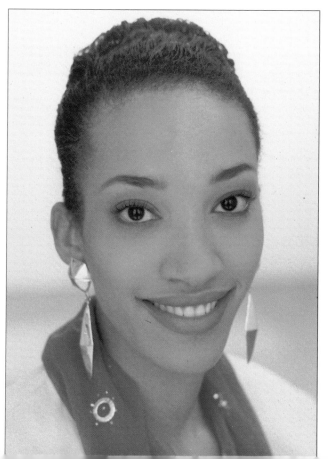

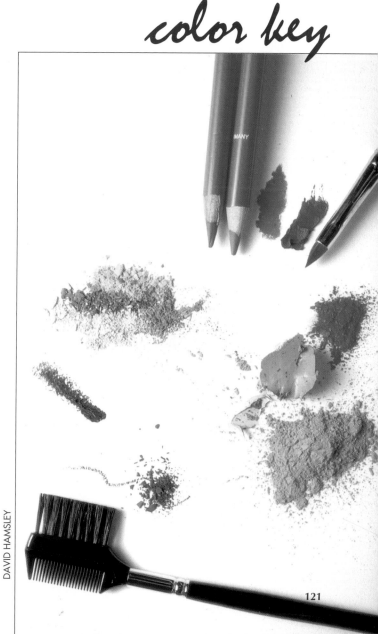

DAVID HAMSLEY

121

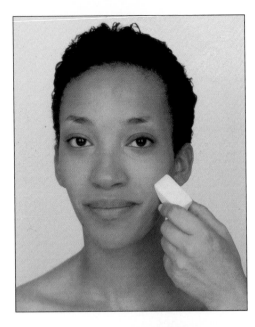

Step 1: Following the application of concealer, soft mocha cream foundation is applied using a wedge to even the skintone.

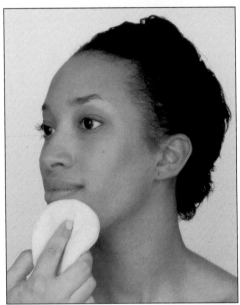

Step 2: Ochre loose powder is pressed onto the face to set the makeup, then buffed with a powder brush to remove excess powder.

Step 3: A selection of peach, yellow, oyster, and persimmon red shadows colors the eye, followed by a fine line of charcoal liner at the base of the lashline; then brows are filled with a soft coal and brown shadow.

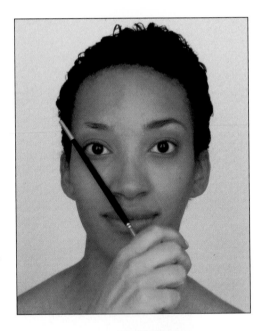

Step 4: Three coats of black mascara are applied to the eyelashes.

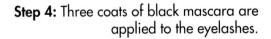

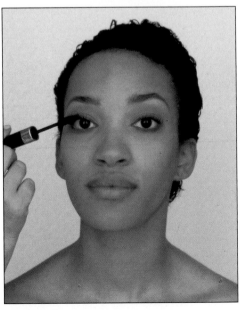

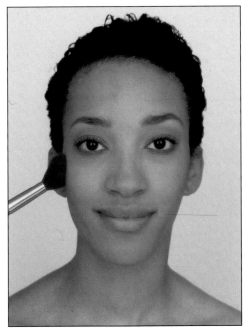

Step 5: Cheeks are gently enhanced with soft persimmon and natural loose powder.

Step 6: Coral pink lipstick is applied using a tapered lip brush.

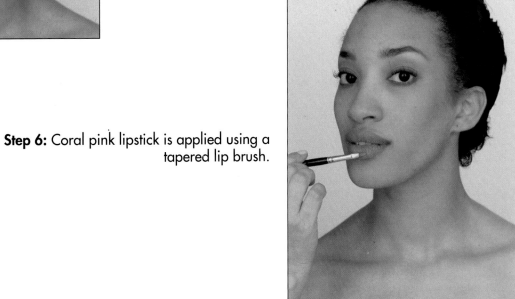

Step 7: To quickly change the makeup to coordinate with an evening dress, eyes are contoured using a deep brown shadow, and lips are filled with a deep matte ginger lipstick.

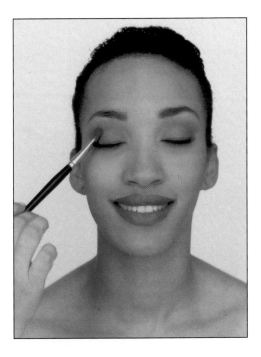

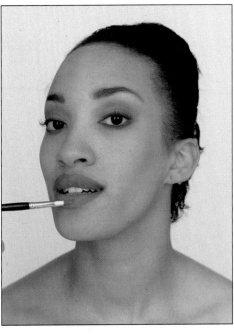

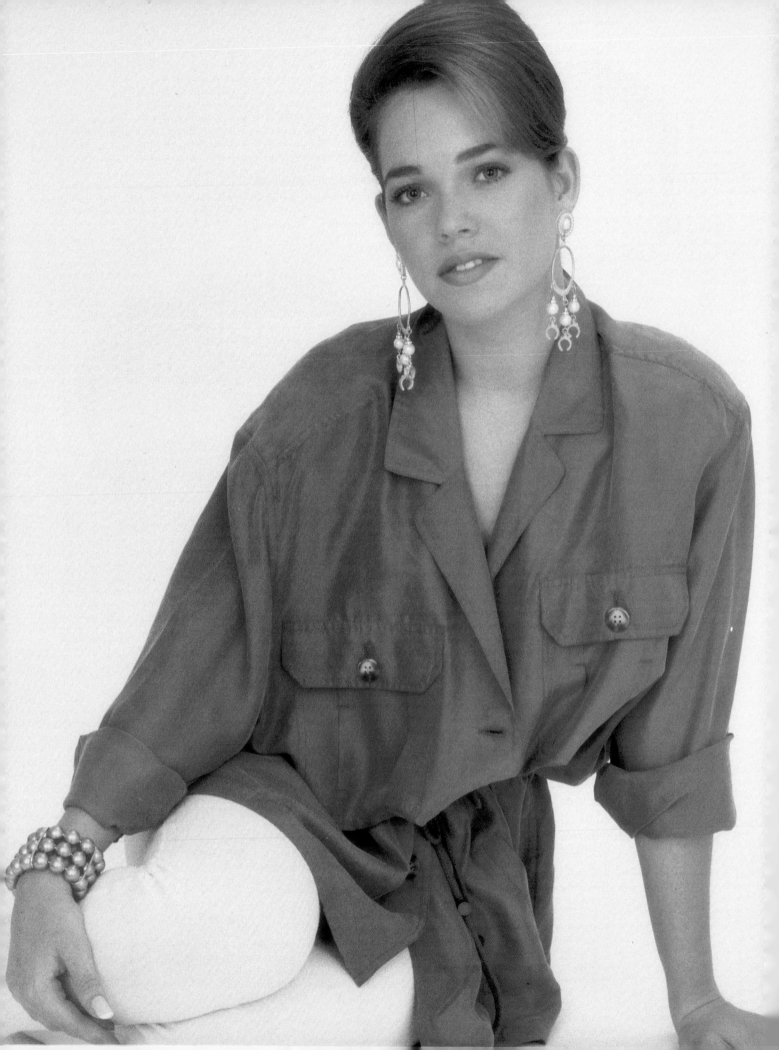

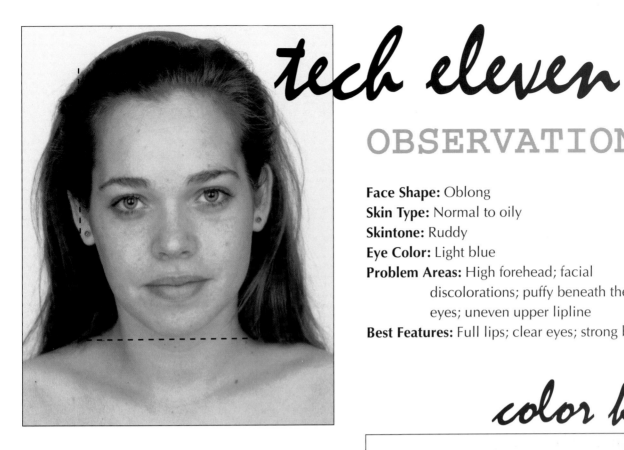

OBSERVATIONS

Face Shape: Oblong
Skin Type: Normal to oily
Skintone: Ruddy
Eye Color: Light blue
Problem Areas: High forehead; facial discolorations; puffy beneath the eyes; uneven upper lipline
Best Features: Full lips; clear eyes; strong brows

Model: Ingrid
Agency: Gilla Roos, New York City
Hair: René/Peter's Place, Great Neck, New York
Makeup: Pamela Taylor. New York City
Accessories: The Accessory Shop, New York City
Photography: Christian Pollard, New York City

color key

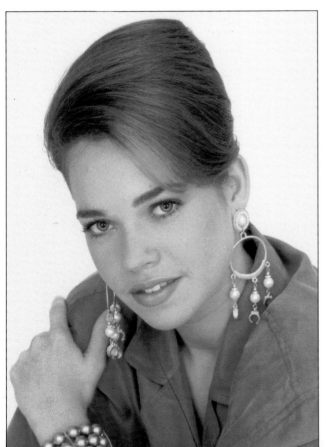

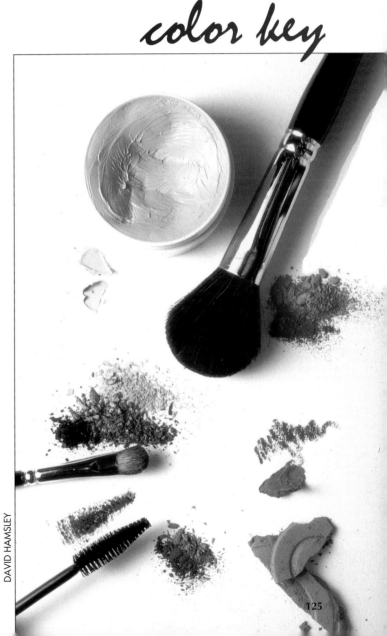

DAVID HAMSLEY

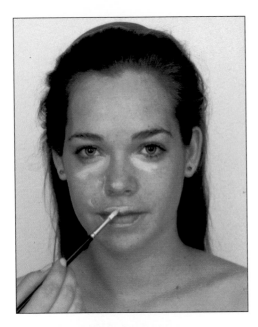

Step 1: Lips, eyes, and facial blemishes are spot concealed to even the area.

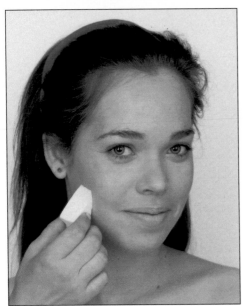

Step 2: Cream foundation applied to a moistened wedge is applied over the entire face.

Step 3: Natural beige loose powder is pressed over the face and neck, then buffed with a powder brush.

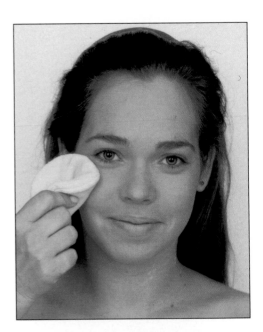

Step 4: Natural peach and soleil blusher is blended and applied to the cheekbones, forehead, and chin.

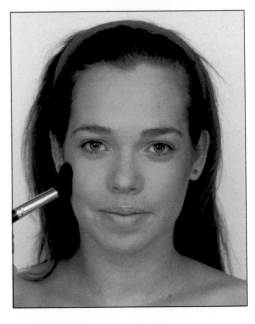

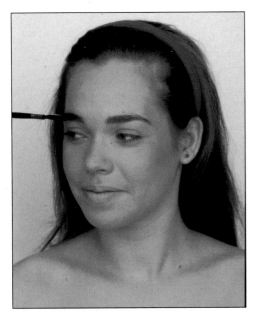

Step 5: Brows are enhanced using light and dark brown shadows, then brushed into shape.

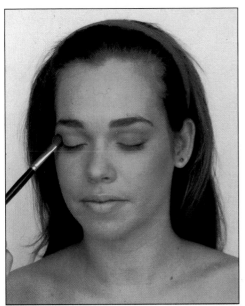

Step 6: Soft pearlized brown and matte yellow shadow is applied to the eyes and blended to soften any hard lines.

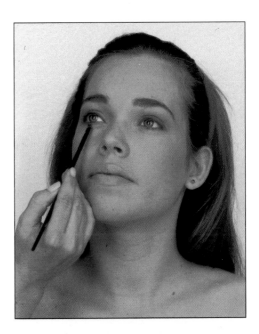

Step 7: Soft black shadow is blended beneath the eyes using an angular brush.

Step 8: Natural soft brown lipliner enhances the lip shape; nutshell brown lipstick is then applied.

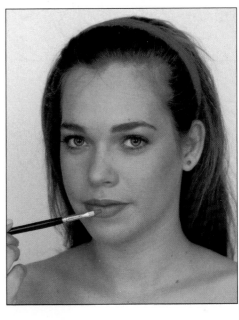

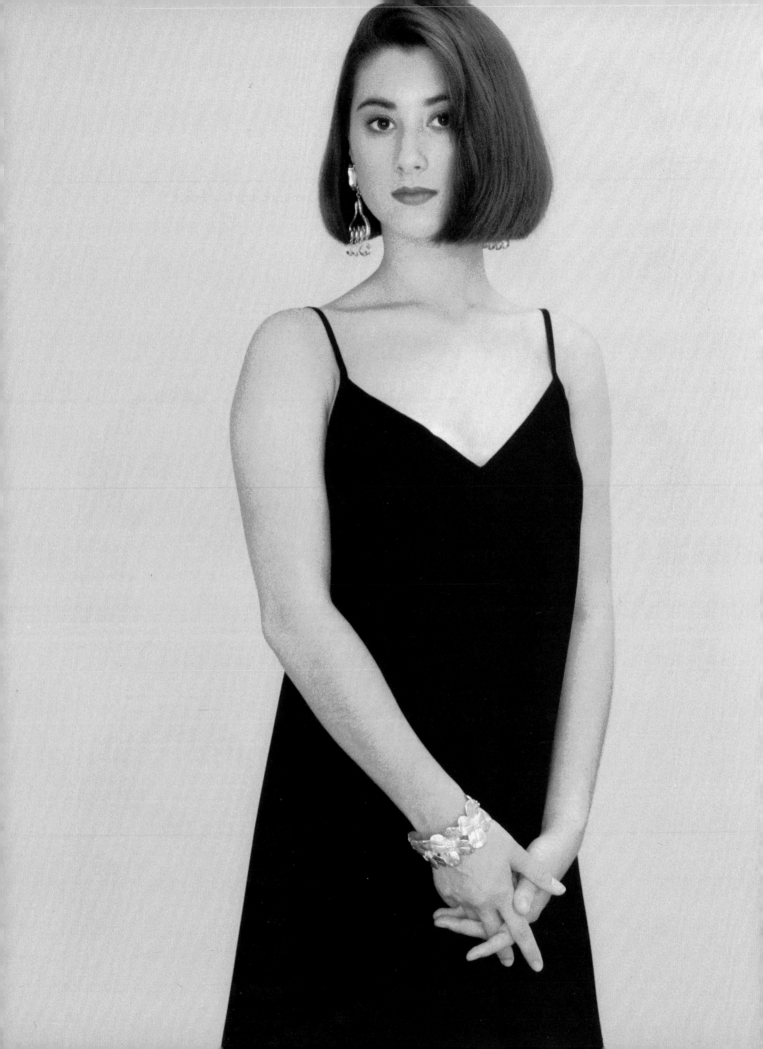

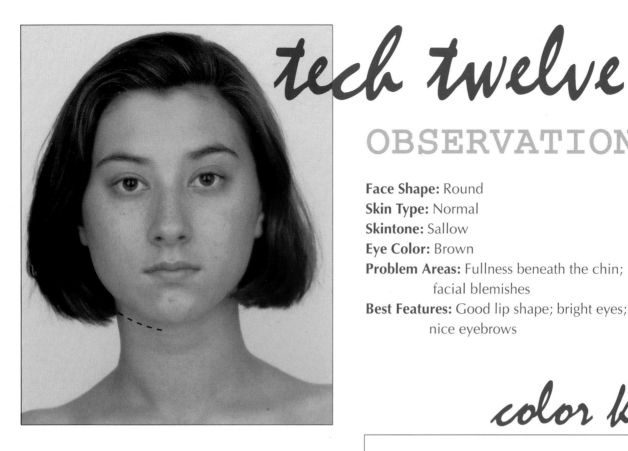

tech twelve
OBSERVATIONS

Face Shape: Round
Skin Type: Normal
Skintone: Sallow
Eye Color: Brown
Problem Areas: Fullness beneath the chin; facial blemishes
Best Features: Good lip shape; bright eyes; nice eyebrows

color key

Model: Jennifer
Hair: Peter Anthony, Nouvelle, Babylon, New York
Makeup: Pamela Taylor, New York City
Photography: Christian Pollard, New York City

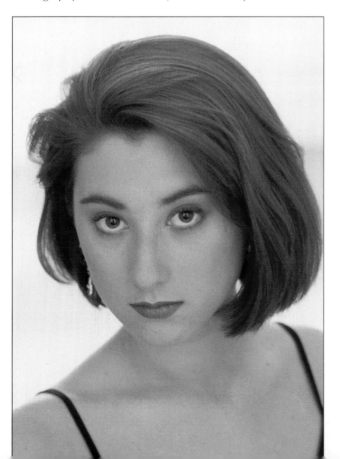

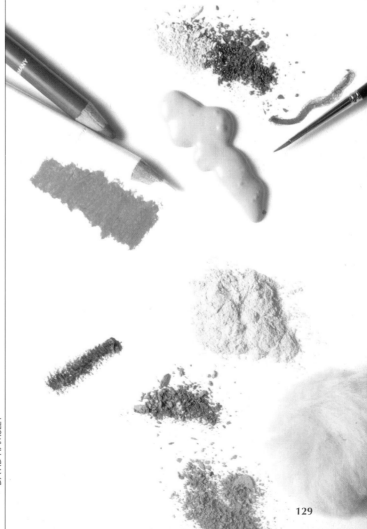

DAVID HAMSLEY

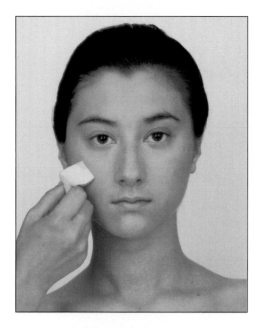

Step 1: After the concealer has been applied, medium beige water-based foundation is applied using a moistened sponge wedge; then the makeup is set with a loose neutral powder.

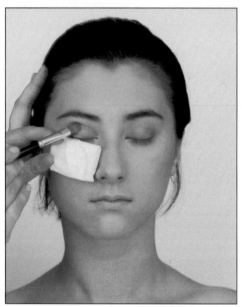

Step 2: Using a tissue beneath the lid, nut-shell pearl and oyster beige shadow is applied to the eyelids.

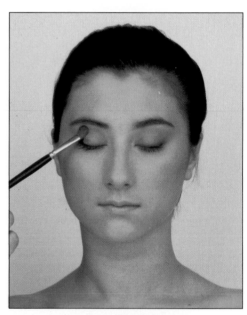

Step 3: After black cake eyeliner is applied, all eye make-up is then blended.

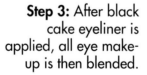

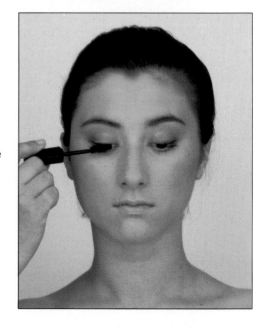

Step 4: Black mascara is applied to the upper and lower lashes.

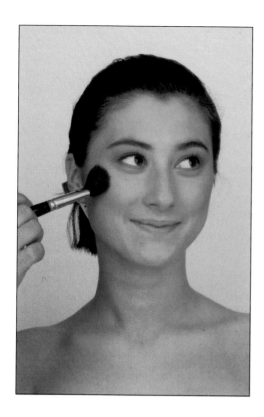

Step 5: Soft peach powdered blush is applied to the cheek area.

Step 6: The natural lipline is outlined with a white pencil to enlarge the lip shape.

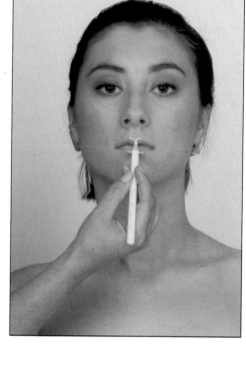

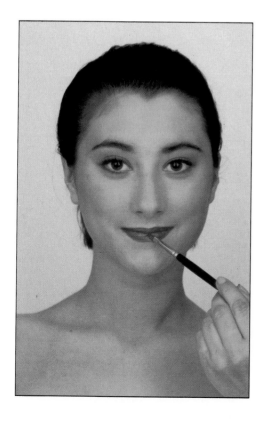

Step 7: Brick lipcolor fills the lip shape; then all makeup is blended.

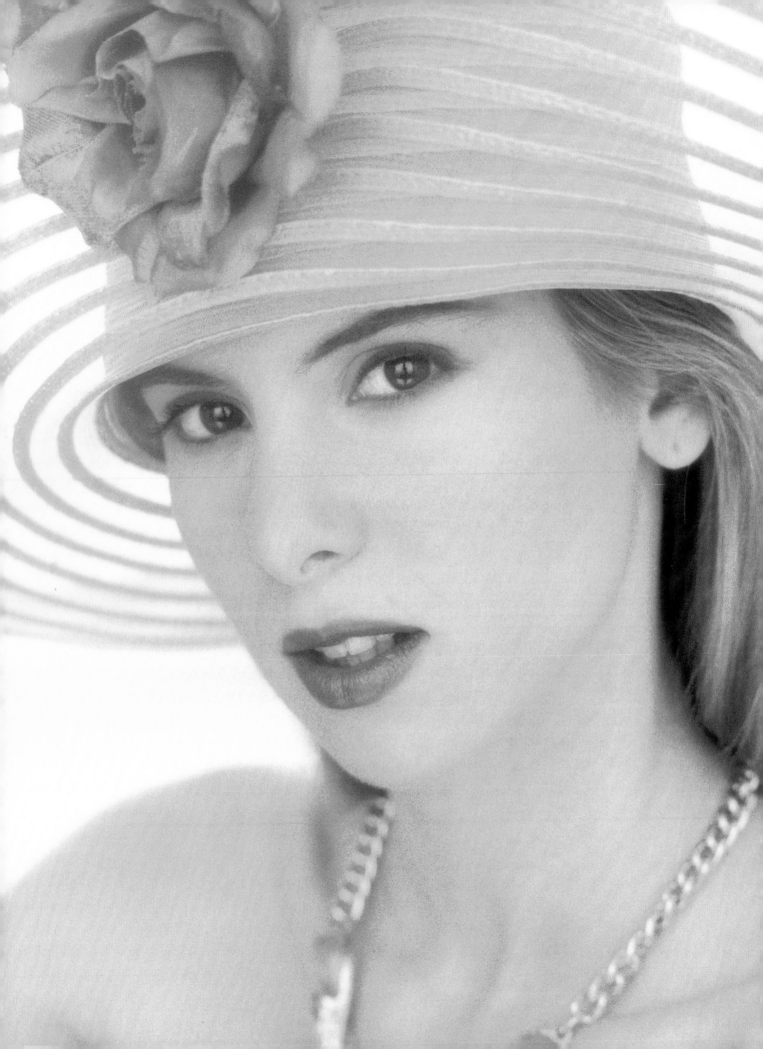

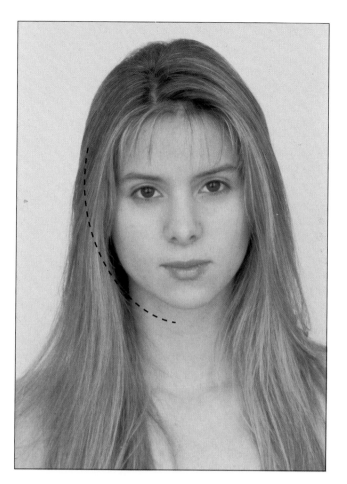

color key

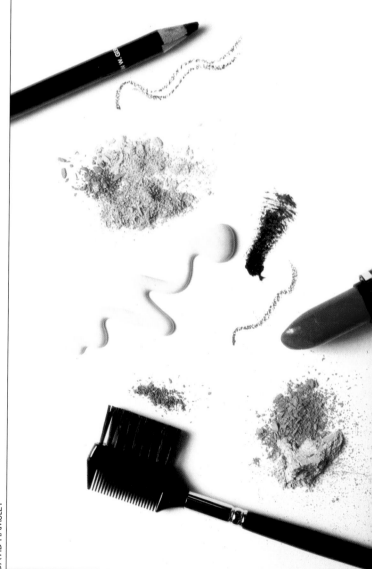

OBSERVATIONS

Face Shape: Oval
Skin Type: Normal to oily
Skintone: Sallow
Eye Color: Brown
Problem Areas: Width at bridge of nose;
      recessed area beneath the eyes
Best Features: Very attractive facial shape;
      full bottom lip; nice eye color.

Model: Sherylann
Agency: Lure, New York City
Makeup: Pamela Taylor, New York City
Accessories: The Accessory Shop, New York City
Photography: Christian Pollard, New York City

DAVID HAMSLEY

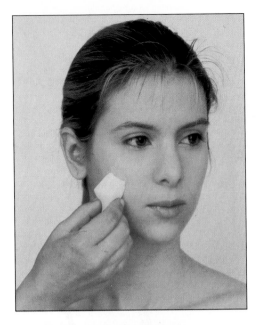

Step 1: Following concealer, liquid foundation is spot blended to even the skintone.

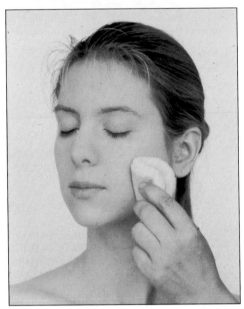

Step 2: Translucent powder sets the base and is pressed on using a velour puff.

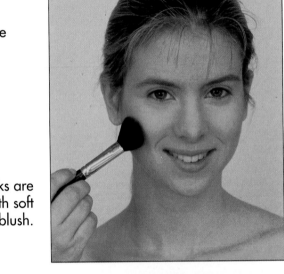

Step 3: Cheeks are enhanced with soft peach powder blush.

Step 4: Brows are enhanced and shaped using an angular brush and an ash powdered shadow.

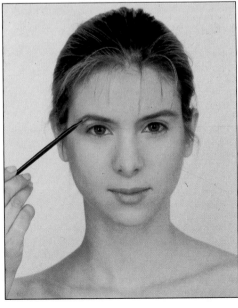

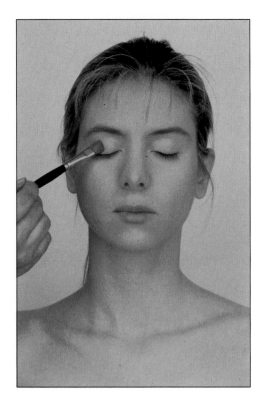

Step 5: Golden yellow shadow is applied to the lids; soft reddish brown shadow is used as a contour shade in the crease.

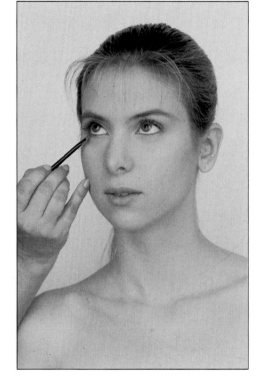

Step 6: Soft reddish brown shadow is tapered into the corners of the lashline beneath the eye using an angular brush, followed by a generous application of black/brown mascara.

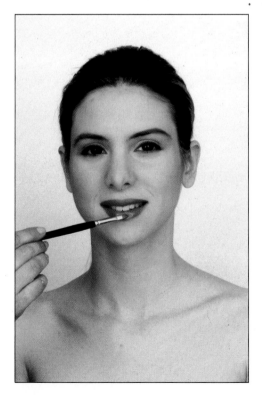

Step 7: Soft red lipliner is applied to the natural lipline and filled with a complementary lip color.

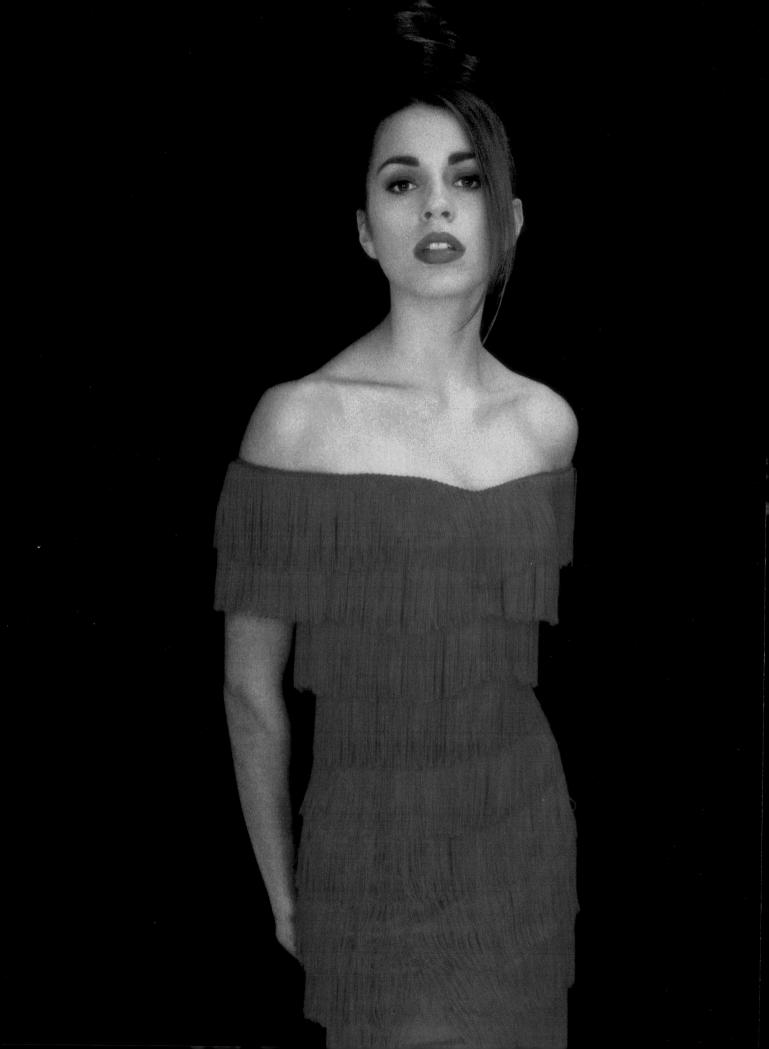

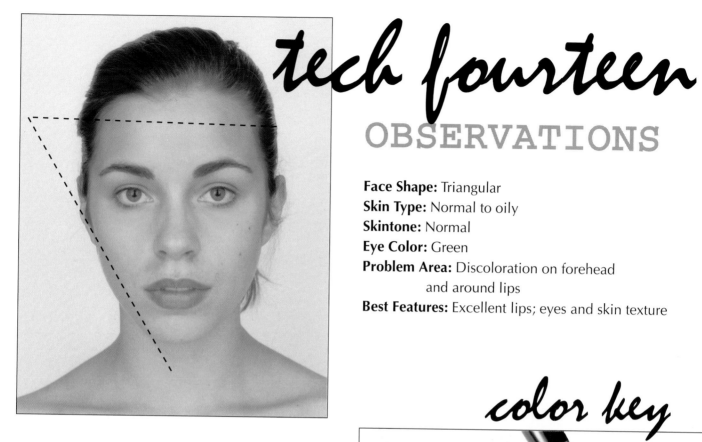

tech fourteen
OBSERVATIONS

Face Shape: Triangular
Skin Type: Normal to oily
Skintone: Normal
Eye Color: Green
Problem Area: Discoloration on forehead
and around lips
Best Features: Excellent lips; eyes and skin texture

color key

Model: Robin
Agency: Boldt, New York City
Hair: José Raphael, New York
Makeup: Pamela Taylor, New York City
Accessories: The Accessory Shop, New York City
Photography: Christian Pollard, New York City

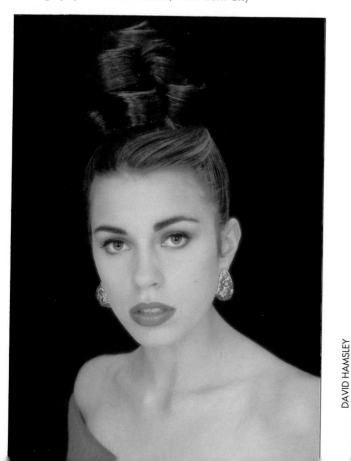

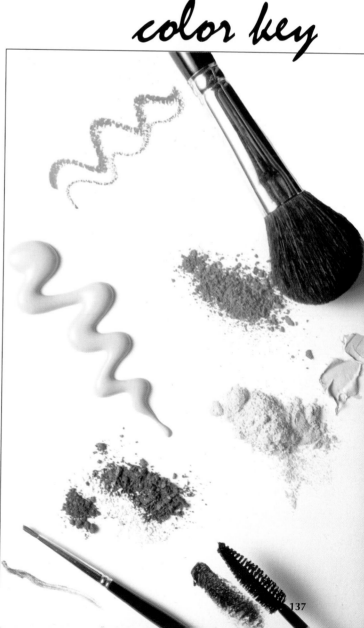

DAVID HAMSLEY

137

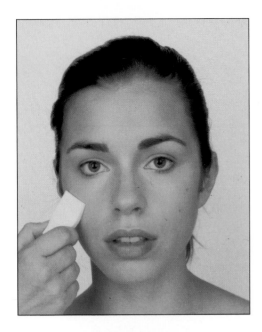

Step 1: Concealer is spot blended using a latex wedge in discolored areas.

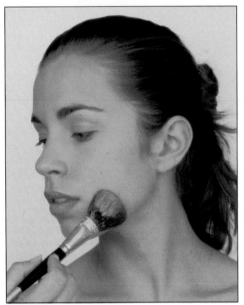

Step 2: After a water-based foundation has been applied, nutshell loose powder is buffed on to set the makeup.

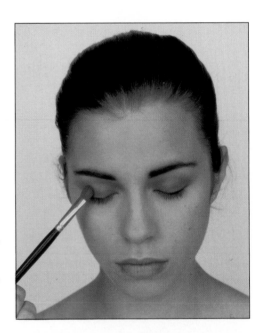

Step 3: Amethyst, cream, and berry shadow is blended onto the lid; the lighter shade is applied beneath the browbone.

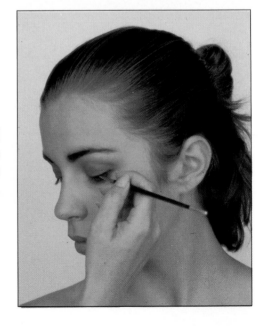

Step 4: Jet black cake eyeliner is applied using a sable liner brush to the lashline and softly shaded at the outer edge of the lower lashline.

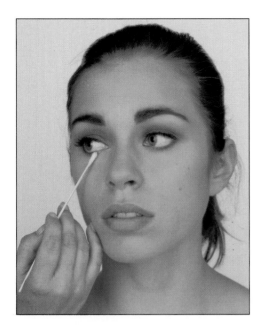

Step 5: A surgical cotton swab is used to soften the line.

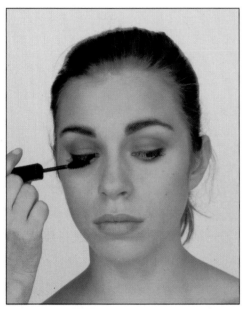

Step 6: Soft black mascara is applied to the upper and lower lashes.

Step 7: A mauve blush is swept over the cheekbones and blended to distribute the color.

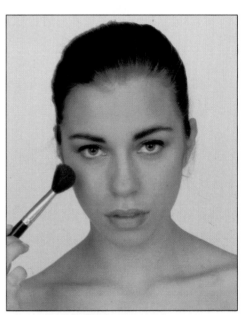

Step 8: Plum lipliner is applied to the outer edge of the natural lipline, then filled using a deep cherry lipstick.

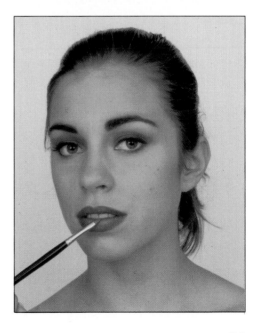

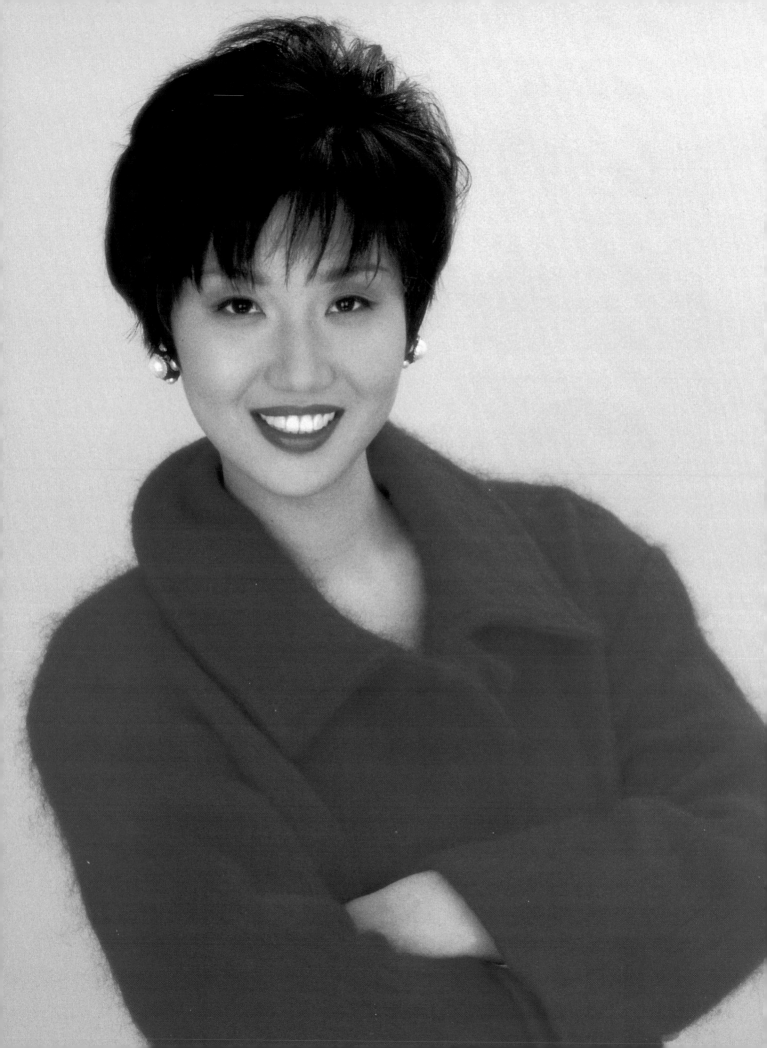

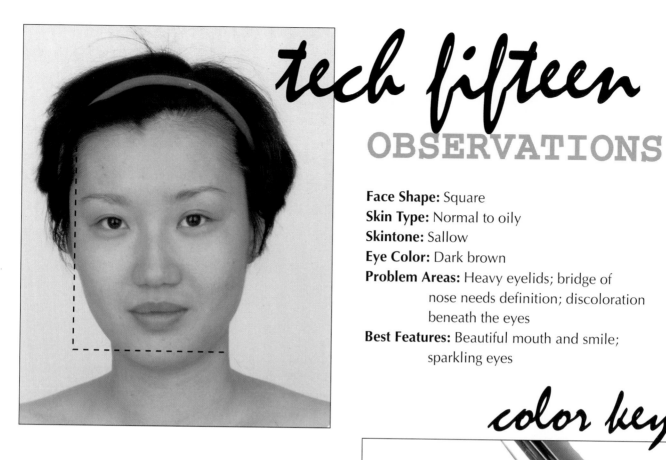

tech fifteen
OBSERVATIONS

Face Shape: Square
Skin Type: Normal to oily
Skintone: Sallow
Eye Color: Dark brown
Problem Areas: Heavy eyelids; bridge of
        nose needs definition; discoloration
        beneath the eyes
Best Features: Beautiful mouth and smile;
        sparkling eyes

color key

Model: Kim
Hair: José Raphael, New York
Makeup: Pamela Taylor, New York City
Accessories: The Accessory Shop, New York City
Photography: Christian Pollard, New York City

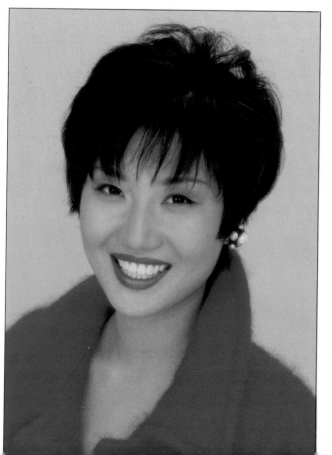

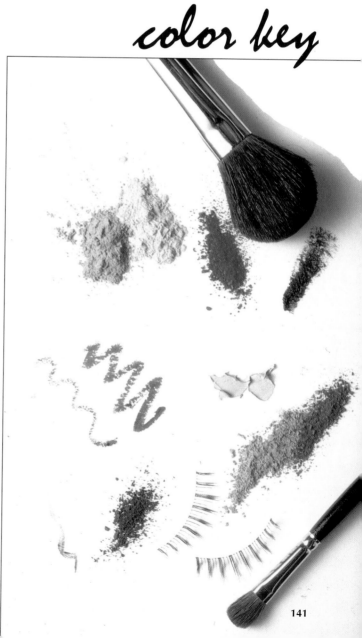

DAVID HAMSLEY

141

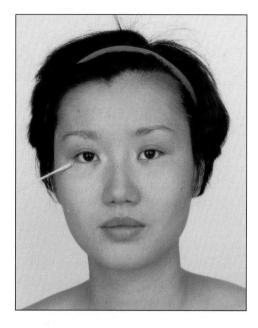

Step 1: Concealer is applied to the discoloration beneath the lower lid, and a deeper shade is added to recede the puffiness.

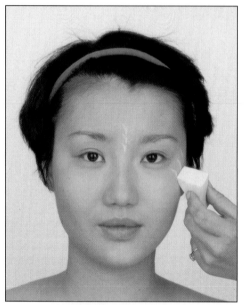

Step 2: After applying cream highlights to the center of the nose and at the height of the cheekbones to bring out the areas, natural and beige water-based foundations are applied to even the skintone.

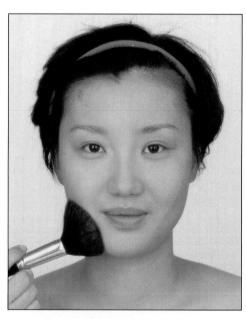

Step 3: Ochre and natural loose powder is buffed on with a powder brush to set the makeup.

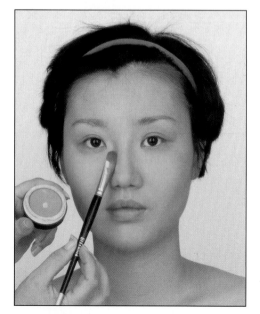

Step 4: An ash brown powdered contour is applied to a tapered brush and applied from the bridge of the nose down the sides of the nostrils to lengthen the nose.

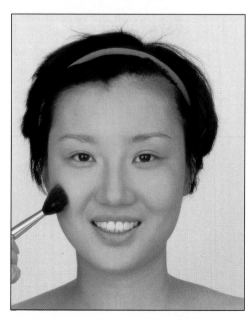

Step 5: Soft red powder blush is applied to the apple of the cheeks and distributed lightly around the face.

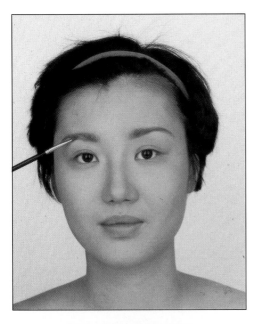

Step 6: Brows are defined using two tones of brown shadow applied with a moistened angular shadow brush.

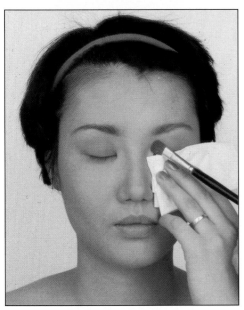

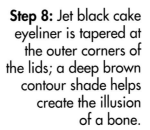

Step 7: A medium matte pumpkin shadow is swept over the entire lid beneath the browbone.

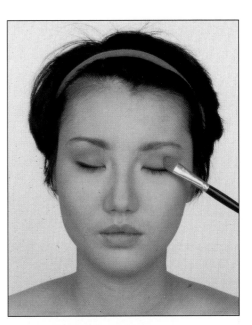

Step 8: Jet black cake eyeliner is tapered at the outer corners of the lids; a deep brown contour shade helps create the illusion of a bone.

Step 9: Red lipsticks are blended to match the outfit and applied to the lips; all makeup is blended well.

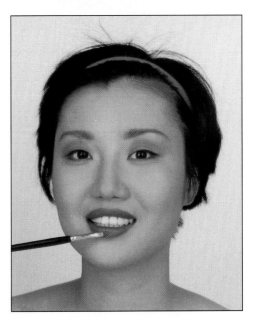

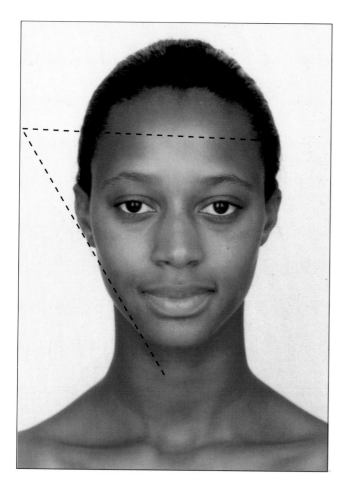

color key

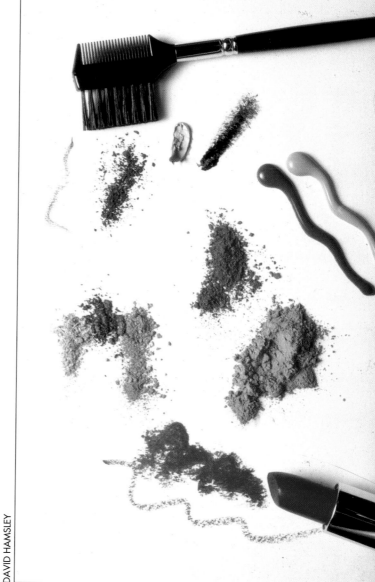

DAVID HAMSLEY

OBSERVATIONS

Face Shape: Triangular
Skin Type: Normal to oily
Skintone: Medium/dark
Eye Color: Dark brown
Problem Areas: Puffy eyelids; mixed skintone;
      sparse eyebrows
Best Features: Beautiful eyes and smile

Model: Lucie
Agency: Gilla Roos, New York City
Hair: Peter Anthony, Nouvelle, New York
Makeup: Pamela Taylor, New York City
Photography: Christian Pollard, New York City

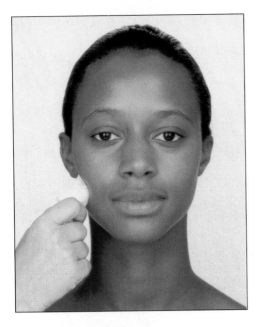

Step 1: Cocoa and yellow concealers are mixed and applied to discolored areas on the face. Next a water-based foundation is blended and applied to even the skintone.

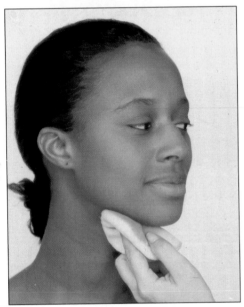

Step 2: Ochre loose powder is pressed onto the face to set the makeup base.

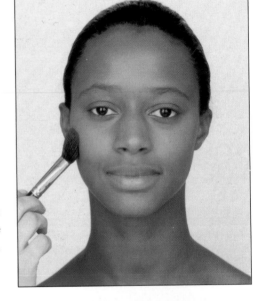

Step 3: A mauve blush is applied to enhance the cheekbones.

Step 4: Brows are arched and shaped with a matte brown/black powder. Next a selection of ginger, peach, and amethyst is carefully applied to the lid and blended.

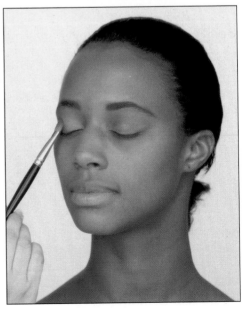

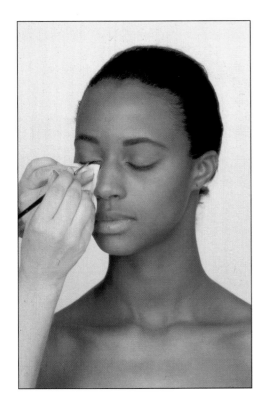

Step 5: A fine line of black cake eyeliner is applied at the base of the lashline.

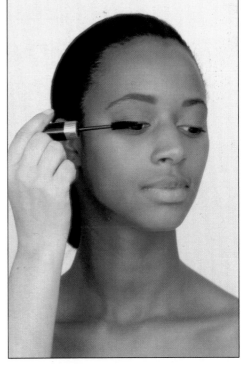

Step 6: Deep brown cake eyeliner is moistened and applied to the base of the upper eyelashes.

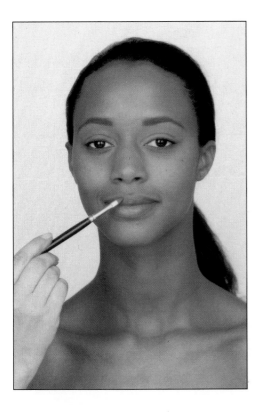

Step 7: Soft rose lipstick is applied to the inner lipline and blended.

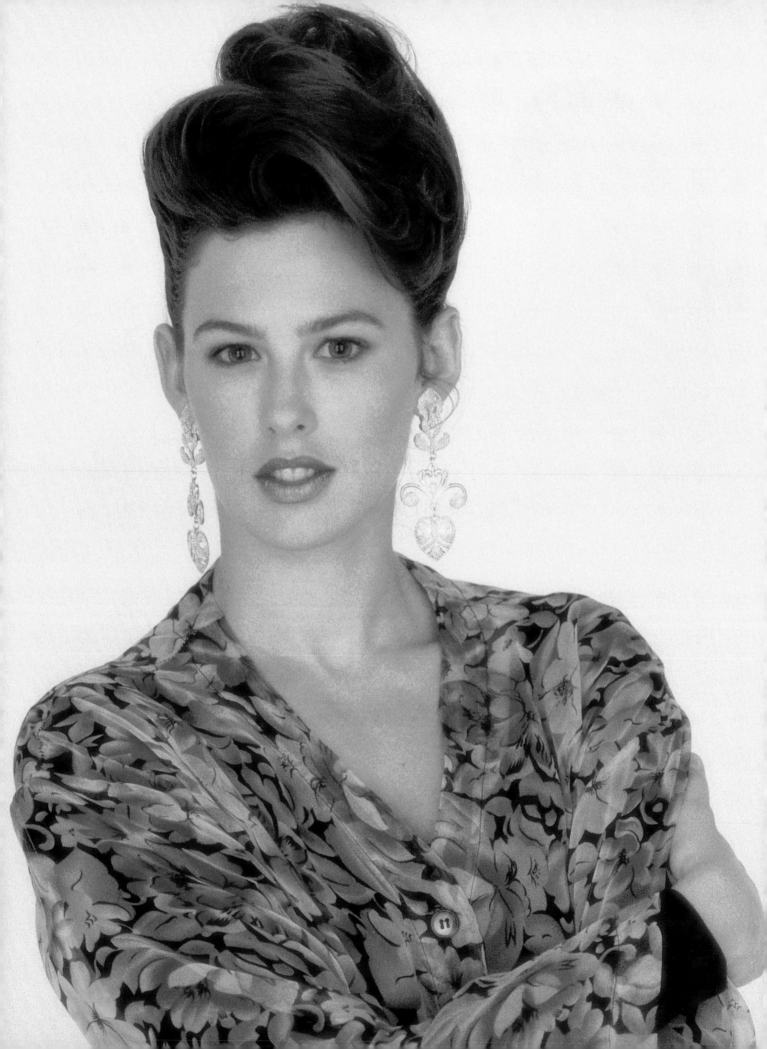

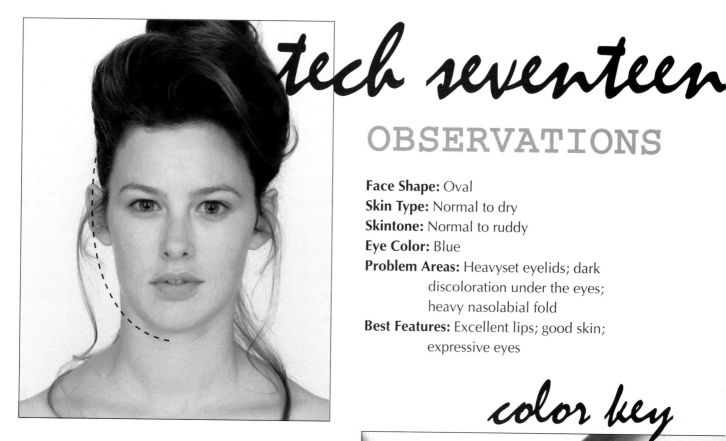

OBSERVATIONS

Face Shape: Oval
Skin Type: Normal to dry
Skintone: Normal to ruddy
Eye Color: Blue
Problem Areas: Heavyset eyelids; dark discoloration under the eyes; heavy nasolabial fold
Best Features: Excellent lips; good skin; expressive eyes

color key

Model: Elan
Agency: Lure, New York City
Hair: René/Peter's Place, Great Neck, New York
Makeup: Pamela Taylor, New York City
Accessories: The Accessory Shop, New York City
Photography: Christian Pollard, New York City

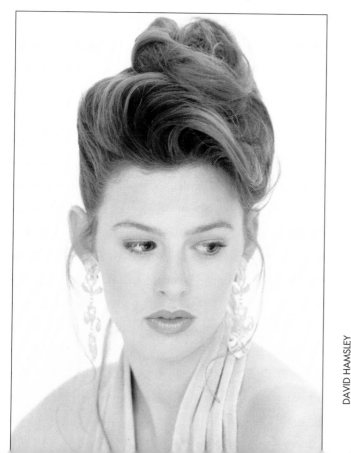

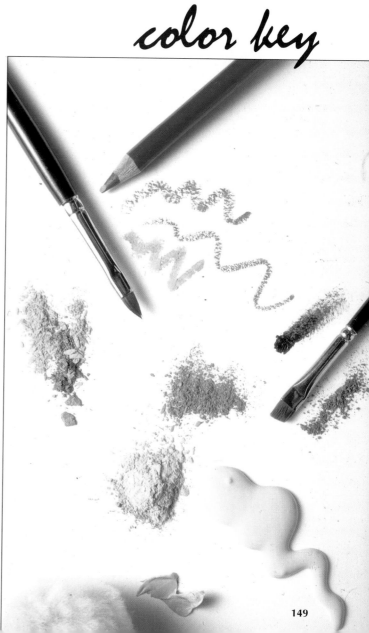

DAVID HAMSLEY

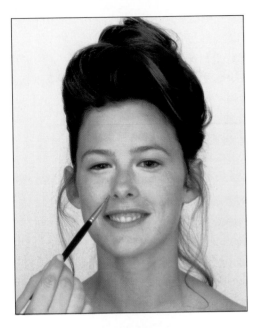

Step 1: Natural and maize concealer is applied to undereye discoloration, and natural concealer is applied into nasolabial fold (laugh lines) to highlight and lift out the recessed area.

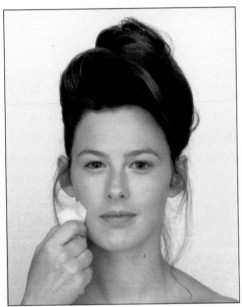

Step 2: Natural water-based foundation is blended onto the face to even the skintone.

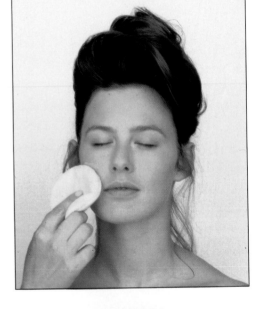

Step 3: Natural beige powders are applied to set the makeup.

Step 4: Pure peach blush is added to the apple of the cheeks to enhance the face.

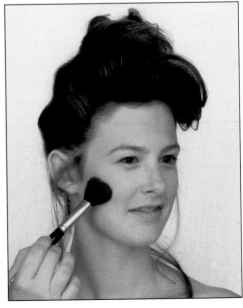

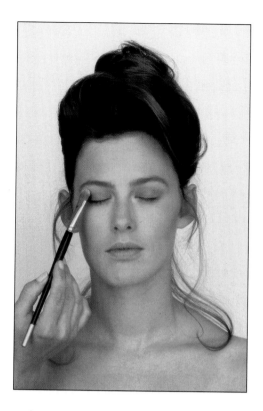

Step 5: Celery green and daffodil yellow shadows are applied to the lid using a sable blender brush; the deeper shade is applied as a contour; the lighter shade as a highlight.

Step 6: Soft celery shadow is moistened and applied beneath the eye using an angular brush; next a generous coat of mascara is applied.

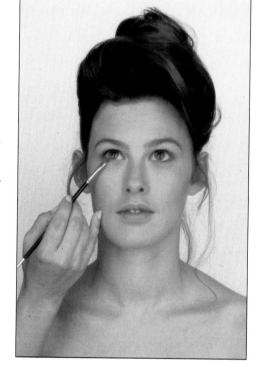

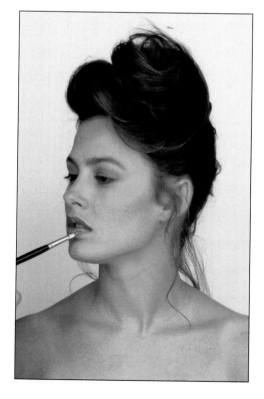

Step 7: Lips are lined using a russet lipliner; next a golden bronze lipstick is blended to fill the lips with color.

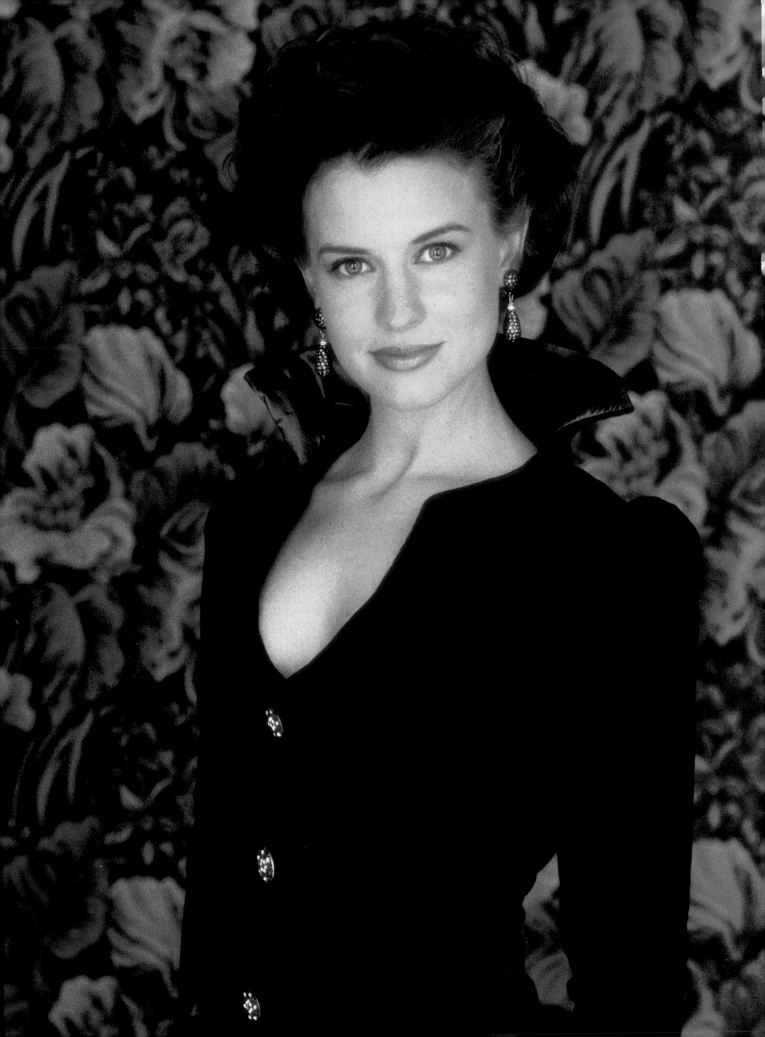

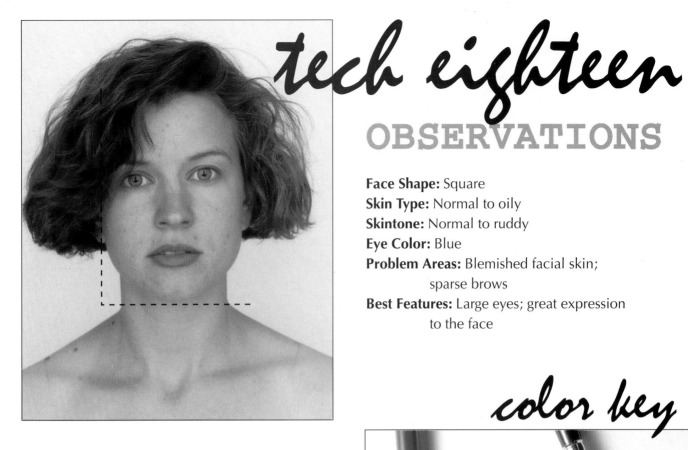

tech eighteen

OBSERVATIONS

Face Shape: Square
Skin Type: Normal to oily
Skintone: Normal to ruddy
Eye Color: Blue
Problem Areas: Blemished facial skin; sparse brows
Best Features: Large eyes; great expression to the face

color key

Model: Karen
Agency: Gilla Roos, New York City
Hair: René/Peter's Place, Great Neck, New York
Makeup: Pamela Taylor, New York City
Accessories: The Accessory Shop, New York City
Photography: Christian Pollard, New York City

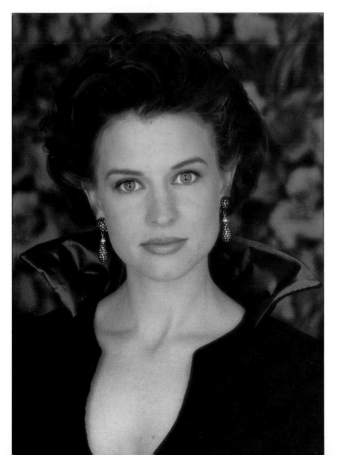

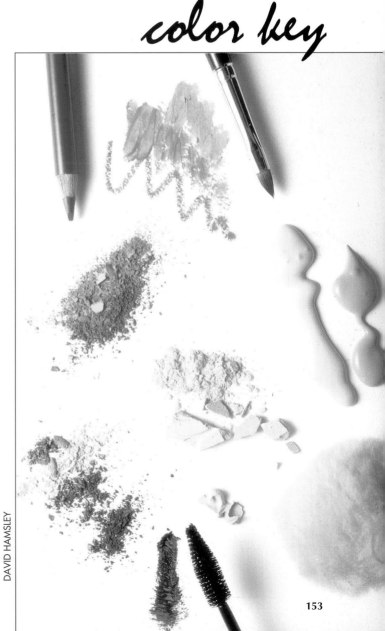

DAVID HAMSLEY

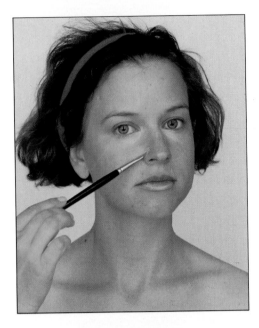

Step 1: Concealer is applied to cover blemishes and discolorations on the face.

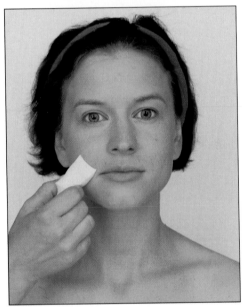

Step 2: Light and medium beige foundation is mixed, then applied using a wedge to even the skintone.

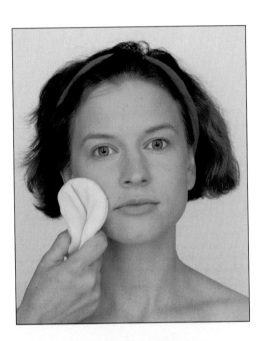

Step 3: Transparent powder is pressed onto the face with a velour puff to set the makeup.

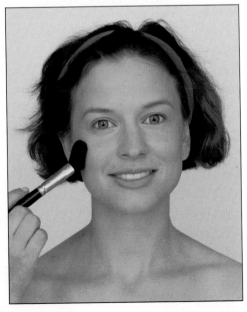

Step 4: Soft peach and bronze blusher is custom blended and applied to the cheeks.

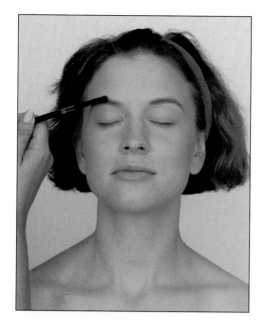

Step 5: Amethyst, berry, soft pink, and celery shadows enhance the lids; then brows are brushed, arched, and shaped.

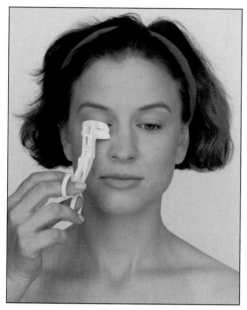

Step 6: Lashes are pressed and curled with a lash curler to lift the lashes.

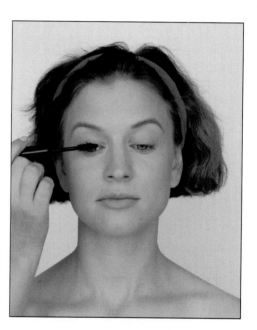

Step 7: A generous coat of mascara is applied to the eyes, followed by a thin line of cake eyeliner.

Step 8: Lips are lined with a mocha lip pencil and filled with a cocoa brown lipstick.

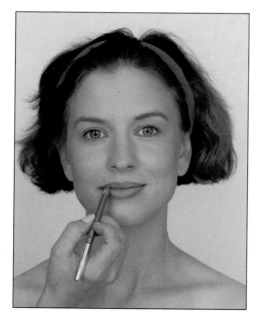

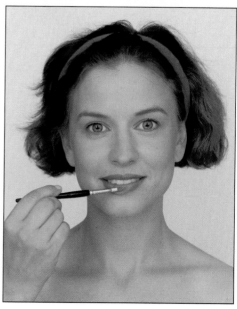

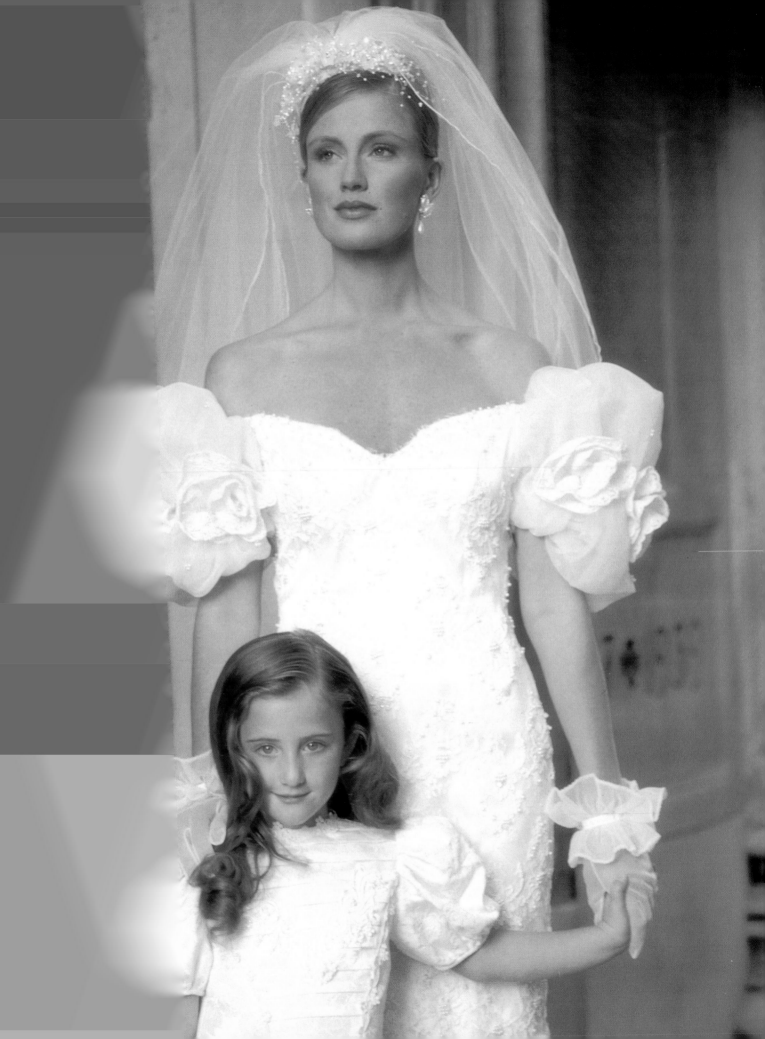

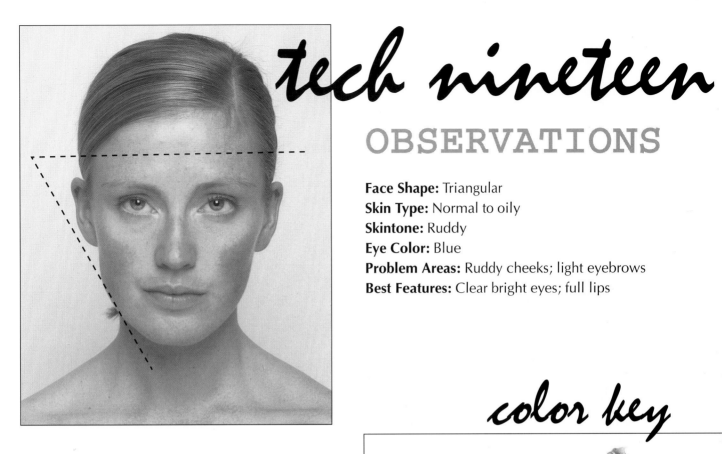

tech nineteen

OBSERVATIONS

Face Shape: Triangular
Skin Type: Normal to oily
Skintone: Ruddy
Eye Color: Blue
Problem Areas: Ruddy cheeks; light eyebrows
Best Features: Clear bright eyes; full lips

Model: Martina (with Meaghan on page 156)
Agency: Zoli, New York City
Ensemble: Bridal Suite, Patchogue, New York
Makeup: Pamela Taylor, New York City
Photography: Kent Squires, New York City

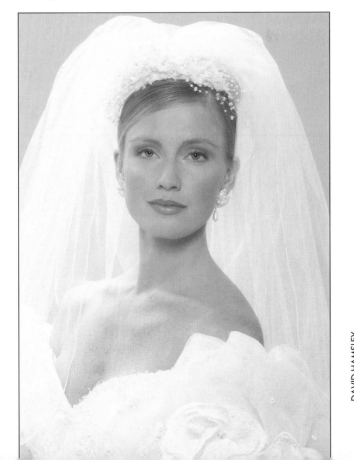

color key

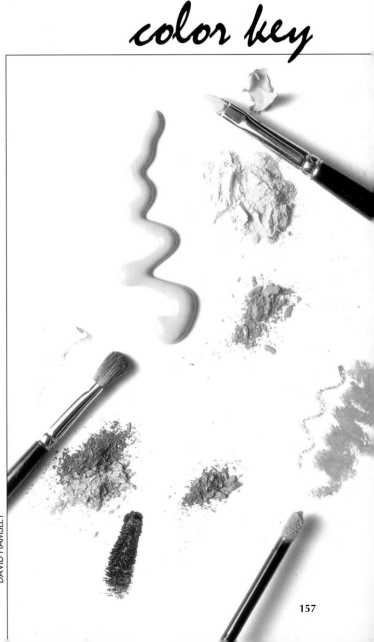

DAVID HAMSLEY

157

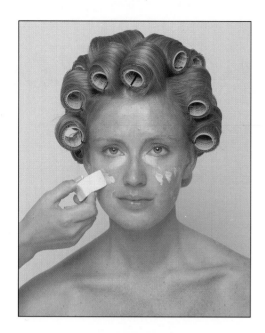

Step 1: To cancel out red, mint color corrector is applied to redness; then concealer is applied to needed areas and lightly blended.

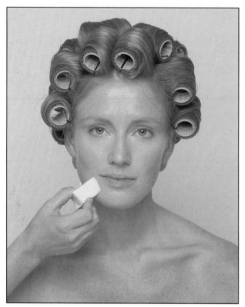

Step 2: Cream makeup is blended over the entire face down into the neckline.

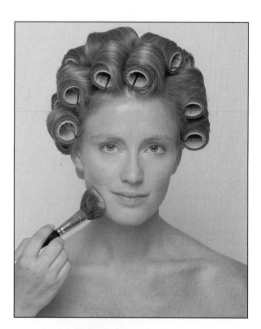

Step 3: Translucent powder is applied to the cream makeup to set the base.

Step 4: Coral cheek color is swept onto the cheekbones and blended.

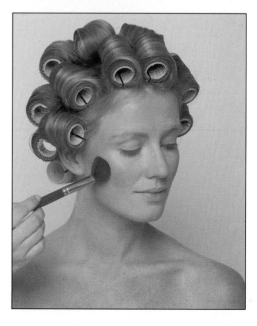

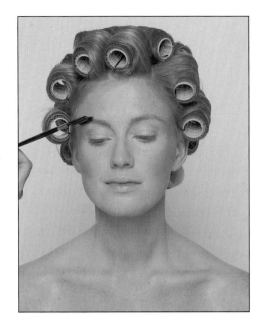

Step 5: Eyebrows are groomed and set with brow-gel.

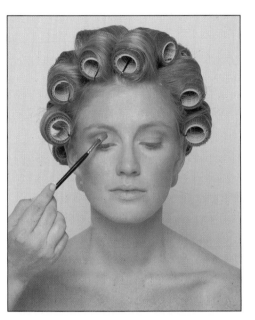

Step 6: Pale peach demi-pearl shadow is applied to the inner eyelid; then soleil matte shadow is blended into the contour.

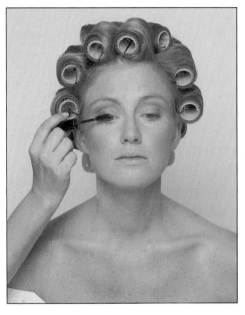

Step 7: Waterproof mascara is carefully applied to the lashes.

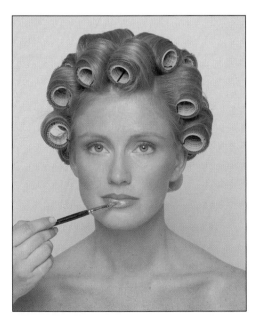

Step 8: Natural lipliner shapes the natural line of the lips; then fresh pink lipstick is added.

editorial makeup

Editorial makeup refers to the type of makeup used in high-fashion magazines. It gives the makeup artist a chance to experiment with color, create new looks, and go beyond the boundaries of the conventional. The artistic aspect of editorial makeup is worth noting because it allows the make-up artist to create a persona for the model. In other words, the photographer or art director wants to convey a certain feeling or theme during a photographic shoot. The makeup artist plays a very big part in establishing the identity or "look" of the model.

This is how one of New York's top fashion photographers describes the role of the makeup artist:

> "The makeup artist establishes an identity for the model through a particular makeup application. The makeup will give the model a certain 'enlightenment' for the images that are going to be produced. The artistic aspect of the makeup application is very important. Most makeup procedures are very prag-matic, step-by-step building blocks. Those are the basics from which to grow. Once you have established all the precedents of doing things adequately and correctly, you are ready to enter the world of creativity."

The basics, of course, include learning proper hand dexteri-ty, base application, and use of color and proper blending. The following editorial photographs are good examples of a finished session. The theme was an androgynous look, so I thickened the model's eyebrows to strengthen her image, but kept her lips full and feminine. The photo shoot took place on top of my studio building in New York City.

(overleaf) ROBERT TRIPICIANO

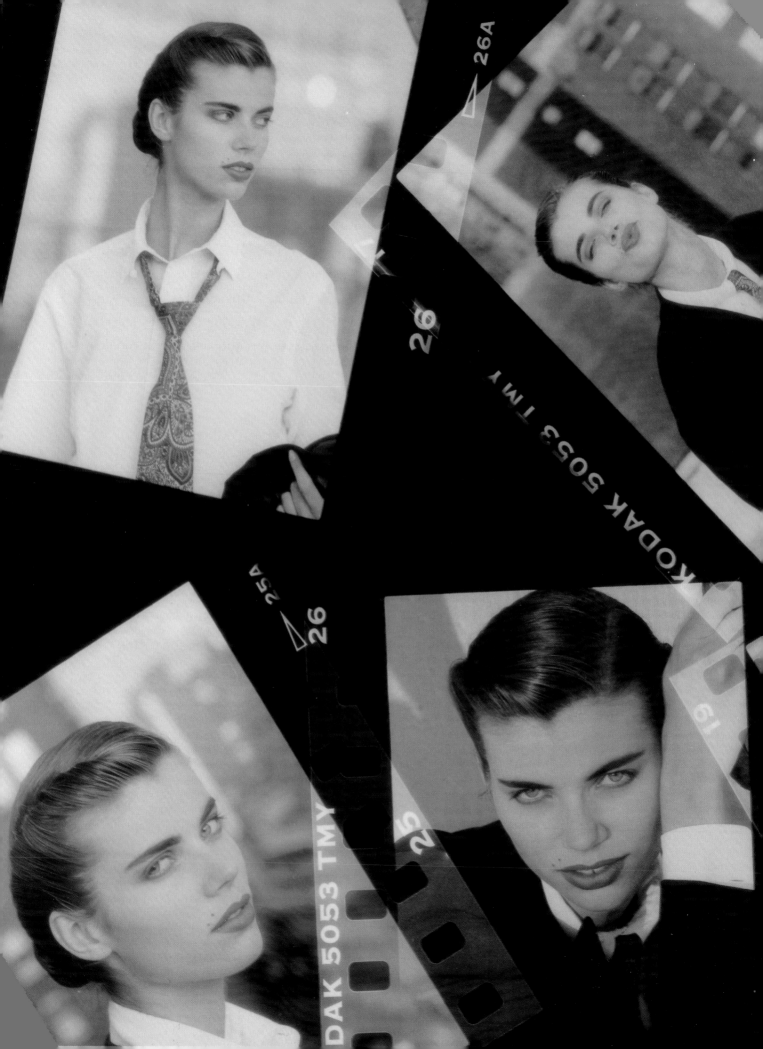

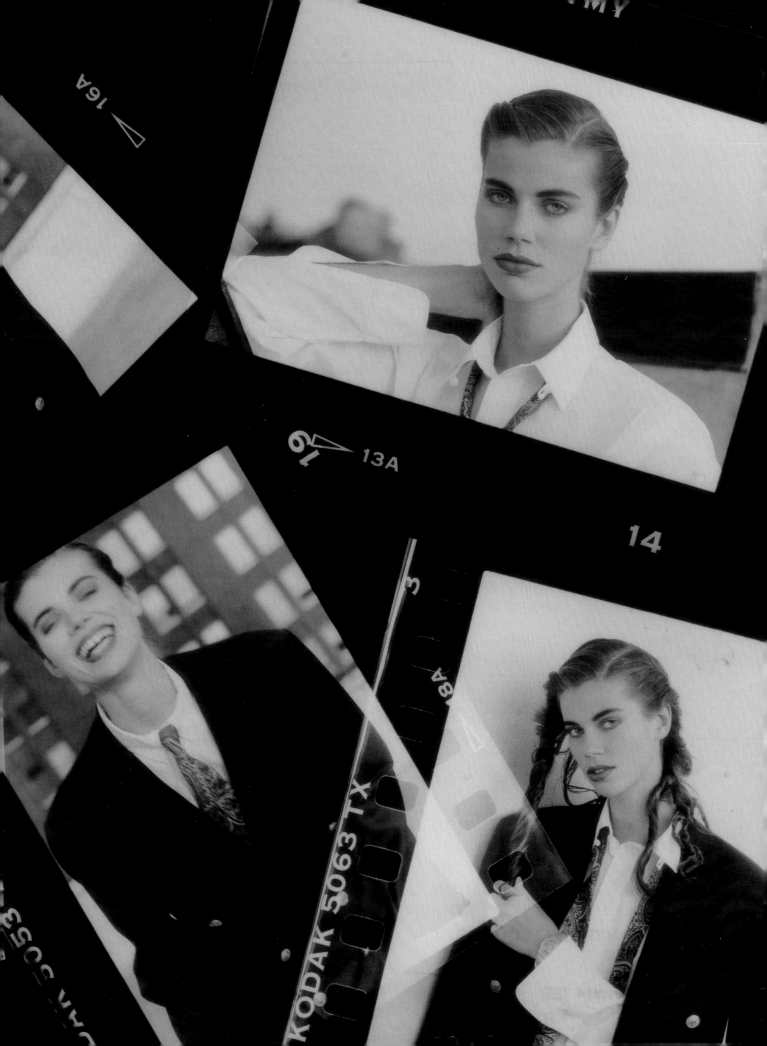

MAKEUP ARTIST NETWORK CLUB

The Makeup Artist Network Club, founded in 1989, is the first professional organization geared for the makeup professional. Learn the latest fashions in makeup styles and industry news. Receive a membership card that entitles you to discounts at professional makeup suppliers and information on upcoming guest events for advanced makeup training and seminars.

For registration information write to:

The Makeup Artist Network Club

119 West 23rd Street, Suite 400

New York, New York 10011

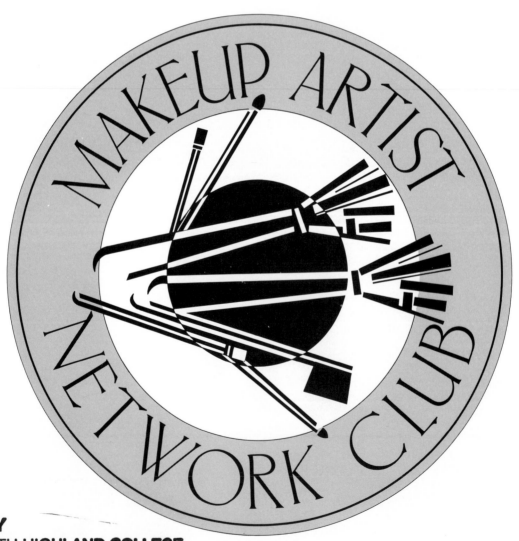